GWYNNE H. DAVIES
N.D., M.N.T.O.S.

Overcoming Food Allergies

HOW TO IDENTIFY AND REMOVE THE CAUSES

You *don't* have to
'live with it'

ASHGROVE PRESS, BATH

Published in Great Britain by
ASHGROVE PRESS LIMITED
Bath Road, Norton St Philip
Bath BA3 6 LW

First published 1985
Fourth printing May 1987
Revised edition February 1989
Reprinted 1990, 1991, 1993
This edition 1996
Reprinted 1998

ISBN 1–85398–088–9

Photoset by Ann Buchan (Typesetters), Middlesex
Printed and bound in Great Britain by
Redwood Books, Trowbridge, Wiltshire

Overcoming Food Allergies

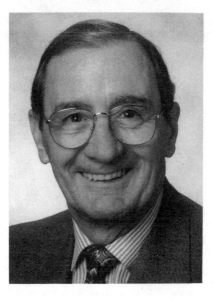

Gwynne H. Davies lives and practices in Taunton, Somerset. After a career in the Fleet Air Arm, he studied Naturopathy and has practised for twenty years, specialising in Clinical Ecology six years ago.

He is a member of the Naturopathic, Osteopathic Society and Register; an Associate of the British Dietetic Association; a Member of the McCarrison Society; a Member of the British Homoeopathic Association; and a Member of the British European Osteopathic Association.

Gwynne Davies has lectured all over England on food allergies.

CONTENTS

Page

All royalties from the
sale of this book will go to the
British Institute for Brain Injured Children

ACKNOWLEDGEMENTS

There are so many people I would like to thank: Terence Williams for his initial encouragement and tutelage and Brian Butler for his invaluable insight and transferrence of knowledge of applied kinesiology; Mike Stewardson for his encouragement and correction of medical terminology; Anne Reilly, my secretary, who has worked so hard and at inconvenient hours to produce a typescript; Kay and Hazel Lazare who worked so hard to produce the research data in a graphical format; Rosemarie for her support and love. Thank you also to my patients who have made this book possible and supported me when enthusiasm or energy flagged.

Thank you all.

INTRODUCTION

Medicine is always in a state of impending uncertainty. The fact we rely on today may be in question by next week. The state of mind of a physician ought to reflect a corresponding humility, to display a measure of open mindedness in face of the overwhelming incompleteness of our knowledge about the living organism, where every step in a new direction, if one is prepared to look in a new direction, reveals a jungle or an abyss rather than an ordered path. All too often, despite the frequently available but clearly unlearnt lessons of the past, when the previous decades' derided nonsense became with monotonous regularity next year's self evident orthodoxy, such preparedness is conspicuous only by its absence. Time and again over the last two hundred years the medical establishment (which, beware, we all have a tendency to rush to join, for we all wish to have our views accepted and once accepted not materially altered) has covered its embarassingly flat-earth thinking by claiming for its own tomorrow the ground it had scorned yesterday. It has done so with breathtaking insolence and often with scant acknowledgement of the territory's pioneers, especially should they have, like the author of this book, the impertinence not to be orthodoxly medically qualified.

This excellent and stimulating book deserves and I trust will receive a careful inspection both from the professional and the non-professional reader. It is skillfully written so as to be useful to the one and accessible to the other.

Clinical ecology, the investigation of the influence of environment in the search for full health, has many aspects. The effect of food allergy or intolerance is one of those more readily grasped by the non-specialist and one of those most directly amenable to investigation and management. For these reasons it offers a way in to clinical ecology for the new reader and an opportunity of initial self-help for the patient who finds his doctors cannot answer his needs. The relationship of food allergy to vitamin and mineral metabolism and heavy metal poisoning, to inhaled toxins such as solvents and domestic gas and to other environmental influences, for example electro-magnetic fields, is a further intriguing area for research. Indeed this research is already well under way. My profession would do well for the future not to dismiss it. And all these are areas which the reader whose interest is fired by Gwynne Davies' book and who feels drawn to enquire further may explore with profit.

During long acquaintance with the author my attitude has developed from initial scepticism to considerable regard. I heard of him in the first place from my patients who, un-relieved of their chronic symptoms by my ultra-orthodox medicine at that time, began to come back, at first timidly and then, as my ears and eyes opened and my disparaging mouth finally agreed to close, with greater confidence of a sym-pathetic hearing, bringing stories of this unusual man and his unusual methods.

However one may question the rationale of a method or fail to see how there is a mechanism by which it can work, one should not disregard, as some dyed-in-the-wool orthodoxists persist in doing, those patients whose lifelong symptoms leave them or whose chronic debilitating disease is arrested or even reversed when, and only when, their diet is investigated by the author. I have in mind the lifelong asthmatic whom I used to see with frightening regularity and for whom I pro-vided repeat prescriptions with even more frightening regu-larity: I saw her last week, about an entirely different matter: she has not taken a tablet nor used an inhaler for over a year. I have in mind the woman of forty whose rheumatoid arthritis progressed remorselessly, despite the current wonder drugs, until I persuaded her against her very sceptical inclinations to go to the author's clinic. These patients and their examples do not need me to speak for them, they speak for themselves — and for the author.

Gwynne Davies does not pretend to have all the answers nor to cure every patient. We and the majority of naturopaths, doctors and other allied professionals interested in the field recognize the complex interrelationships between this and the other areas of clinical ecology to which I have referred, and between the whole subject and other disciplines such as homoeopathy, acupuncture and osteopathy. For as long as we go on enquiring we continue growing; as we continue to grow we come, however gradually, to a greater understanding. But the more we think we understand the more humble we should try to remain.

MICHAEL STEWARDSON
M.B., B.Chir.

CHAPTER 1

What is Allergy?

The word allergy is often used loosely: people are said to be allergic to anything which does not agree with them. From this has grown the metaphorical or jokey sense in which we speak of a lazy person being 'allergic' to hard work. The true meaning of allergy is more precise: it is a condition in which a person's immune system regards an ordinarily harmless substance as a dangerous 'invader' and responds to it by producing antibodies which in their turn give rise to some unpleasant reactions.

Asthma, eczema and hay fever are perhaps the best known manifestations of allergic reaction, but in fact the full range of reactions is much more devious and complicated. Immunologists work mainly on the basis that extraneous elements such as animal dander, house dust mite, pollens, spores etc., cause an allergic response. I hope to show in this book that, while many people are clearly affected by such substances, their reactions are often caused by a basic food ingestion 'trigger' which provides a breeding ground for those extraneous reactions.

Let me explain in as uncomplicated a way as possible the General Adaptation Syndrome, described fully by Professor Hans Selye of Montreal and adapted and used by Theron Randolph as the Specific Adaptation Syndrome in his book *Human Ecology and Susceptibility to the Chemical Environment*. There are three stages.

1

Stage I.

Alarm reaction – this could be experienced in a number of ways but a typical reaction would be of a child vomiting when fed cows milk. The mother assumes that this is purely an upset tummy and continues to feed the child cows milk. This initial response although significant is ignored and the child then moves into the next stage.

Stage II

This is the stage of adaptation where although toxins (poisons) are being ingested the body shows only minor reactions and the adrenal glands situated on top of the kidneys (see diagram p. 13) are able to cope, producing enough adrenalin and cortisone to keep the system stable. Over the weeks, months or years, depending on the amounts ingested, the adrenal glands slowly shrink to the size of a hazel nut and the toxins begin to win the battle.

Stage III

This is the stage of exhaustion. The adrenal glands are unable to cope, the mast cells discharge their histamine and other chemicals and a severe reaction occurs. This could take the form of an asthma attack, epileptiform convulsion or a skin rash.

It is in these circumstances, when a toxin is ingested, that a pancreatic maladaption takes place and 'triggers' the whole process.

When this stage is reached the extraneous substances have their effect. When in Stage III you might stroke a cat or dog and the eyes might water or you might start sneezing.

A young lad we shall call John came to see me with an asthmatic condition. This was more or less permanent from a

2

youngster and the thing that made it more aggravating was that for as long as he could remember he had always wanted to be a jockey. He adored horses but woe betide him if he went near one. His eyes would stream, his nose would run and his breathing became laboured. I explained to John and his parents about the basic 'trigger' allergen and tested John. He was allergic to milk and white flour and after three weeks of elimination diet, excluding all toxins, he was able to ride a horse with no ill effects at all. As far as I know he is still riding today.

I am not suggesting that all ills are caused by allergic reaction; they certainly are not, and there is no such thing as the complete panacea. But the evidence I have amassed over the years, testing thousands of patients, confirms that the cause of many illnesses, where no physical abnormality can be found, illnesses which defy normal investigatory procedures such as X-Ray, barium meal or enema, or exploratory operation, could be an allergic reaction created by a pancreatic maladaption.

WHAT ARE THE MOST COMMON ALLERGY REACTIONS?

Nasal Catarrh and hay fever

Sometimes these are all year round complaints, although in most cases they are restricted to the months May to September. They differ from the common cold in that the mucous tends to be thin and watery, the eyes become red and irritable, and sneezing bouts are lengthy. Anti-histamine drugs are usually effectively prescribed as suppressants but they have the unfortunate side effect of producing drowsiness and an inability to concentrate.

Asthma and bronchial congestion

This is a distressing condition which causes sufferers a great deal of alarm since they find it impossible to breathe properly. They wheeze and have the sensation of a tight band around chest and throat. This is due to inflammation of the bronchii producing a muscular spasm, an effect that could be likened to cramp in the leg. The frequent association of asthma attacks with stress gives the impression that the asthma is a result of external stress. My findings are the opposite and certainly indicate that the stressor is internal, an allergen. This reduces the adrenal glands into a Stage III (exhaustion) condition and makes them unable to cope with the external stress when it is present.

Eczema, dermatitis, psoriasis

In this painful group of ailments the skin is subject to extreme irritation. Scratching can cause bleeding and inflammation which frequently leads to infection. I hear so often from patients that they have been told they will grow out of this condition, that they need only apply some ointment to calm the irritation and it will go away. The ointment is usually a cortisone based salve which may have the deleterious effect of thinning skin tissues and being absorbed into the system. It is completely fallacious to suggest that one grows out of these things. What in fact happens is that the particular set of mast cells under attack is so weakened that the toxins move on to another set of cells and a different condition is experienced. Hundreds of asthmatics have told me that they had eczema when they were children but they 'grew out of it'. Why then do they have asthma?

Spastic colon, ulcerative colitis, bloating, bowel cramps

Symptoms include intermittent constipation and diarrhoea, soreness of the anus, pains in the lower gut which are often excruciating and a feeling that food goes straight through the system. There may be a bloated feeling after having only a light meal. The subject is unable to eat a normal meal because 'it feels as if I have a lump in my throat', frequently diagnosed as hiatus hernia. I treated a young woman teacher recently who had continual diarrhoea which left her worn out, an urticarial rash (wheals and hives) and nausea all the time. I found she was allergic to many foods, but in particular to wheat. Since eliminating these foods she is now free of symptoms and has returned to teaching. She had previously had three courses of antibiotics but the condition had persisted.

Headache and migraine

Unless you have experienced migraine headache you will find it hard to imagine the awful pain and nausea it entails. Sufferers speak of feeling as though the skull were subjected to terrific forces which threaten either to pull it apart or to crush it to pieces. One young man used to have a twice weekly attack which would paralyse the right side of his body. On the elimination of his allergenic foods he spent forty eight hours completely paralysed and in extreme pain. After this he got up feeling rather washed out. That was two years ago. Since then, I am glad to say, he has had no further attacks. There is usually more than one allergen in these cases.

Genito urinary complaints

These include frequency of micturition (urination) and cystitis without evidence of infection; frigidity; impotence; prostatitis; menstrual disorders; pre-menstrual tension (when the poor woman becomes depressed and irritable, skin lesions appear, the breasts become swollen and sore, and there are pains in the lower abdomen); intra–cyclical bleeding. How pleasant it is to hear my female patients say, 'I had a period and I was not even aware of it starting'.

5

Rheumatism and arthritis

I firmly believe that most cases of arthritis are caused by allergies to food. Thousands of people leading a normal life today are the living proof that ingestants are a key to this dreadful, crippling condition. (see Chapter 3, page 45 for more detail.)

Mental conditions

These can manifest themselves in a whole variety of symptoms: panic attacks and chronic anxiety; depression; hypomania; hyperkinesis; purposeless violence; tension; thought disorder; alcoholism; drug addiction; lack of concentration; epilepsy; dyslexia.

I can hear you saying, ¦there is nothing left, he *does* claim that all conditions can be ameliorated by removing allergenic substances'. Not at all; what I do say is that cases of all these conditions can and have been treated successfully: there is overwhelming evidence to this effect. There are obviously cases of physical and organic collapse that can only be treated by medical treatment or operational procedures, but the fact is that most of these conditions are degenerative over a considerable length of time. Were they treated in the early stages by the elimination of toxic substances from the diet, then thousands of people need not reach that stage. There is an alternative.

It is no coincidence that rarely a day has gone by in recent years without some mention of allergic reaction, whether in newspapers, magazines, on radio or television. A patient of mine recently wrote three episodes of the T.V. nursing series *Angels*, centred on allergies, after she discovered that her own problems were caused by allergens. It is generally held that three to four people in ten suffer from an allergy complaint. At the same time there is no concensus as to why this should be. My suggestion is that we are expecting too much from our bodies in evolutionary terms. We have not had time to adapt to the onslaught of chemical contaminants and additives which

6

are now prevalent in modern food manufacture. If an engine is required to run on a new type of fuel then its component parts must be structurally altered to cope with that fuel. We, however, lack the capacity for drastic internal change. The body would need to go through the slow evolutionary process of millennia in order to achieve such alteration. Meanwhile the food manufacturers get richer and their customers become progressively less healthy. It is a horrifying thought than on average we each consume between 3 and 4 lbs of additives and preservatives per year, on top of which the average annual intake of sugar amounts to 125 lbs per person. Poor pancreas!

THE MECHANISM OF ALLERGIC REACTION

I will now attempt to clarify the mechanism of allergic reaction. A person who is allergic will react to his or her allergen in rather the same way as healthy people react to a possibly dangerous micro-organism or to a poison. In both cases the body's defences are stimulated by the presence of an antigen (living or organic matter foreign to our own proteins). Viruses and bacteria are antigens, and so are normally less dangerous substances like food, pollens etc. Our defences depend on lymphocytes (white cells), whose function it is to distinguish between harmful and innocuous antigens.

When white cells come across an antigen which looks as though it may cause harm to the body they produce anti-bodies; the anti-bodies combine with the antigen and render it harmless. Even in a healthy person it may take several days for the white cells to produce enough anti-bodies to inactivate the antigen, but once the antigen has been dealt with the body has long lasting protection against it. This is the reason why most people only suffer from infectious diseases like measles or chickenpox once in their lives. When the virus attacks for a second time there are anti-bodies at hand to dispose of it quickly. This is the general idea behind vaccination: you are given a minute dose of an antigen which is not strong enough to give you the disease, but is enough to cause the white cells to produce anti-bodies and protect you.

In an allergy-prone person the white cells react to a harmless antigen as if it were an invader. No one is really clear as to why this should happen, although evidence indicates that it may well be a hereditary problem. Allergies do tend to run in families, and there is some evidence that allergic people lack a particular type of white cell which controls the production of anti-bodies. It happens in far too many cases where children have been weaned off the breast too early in their lives, laying them open to infection at a later stage. This often reveals itself as an allergy to dairy products. This tendency is further complicated by the fact that we have not one mechanism for allergic reaction, but several.

What usually happens?

The arrival of an antigen stimulates the production of large quantities of white cells and no particular reaction is noticeable. The anti-bodies, which then have nothing to do but wait for the next invasion, attach themselves to tissue cells known as mast cells. A mast cell contains a number of natural chemicals, histamine being the mot plentiful. The function of the histamine is to increase the flow of fluids in and out of blood vessels, to control the production of fluid in the mucous glands, and to make muscles in the internal organs contract. These events are happening all the time and are regulated automatically by the body without any conscious thought on our part. Once a mast cell has been coated with anti-bodies it is liable to become excited; the next dose of an antigen stimulates the anti-bodies into action and the mast cell reacts by releasing its stock of histamine and other chemicals.

What happens then?

That depends on where the mast cells are located. We are compartmentalised like a ship, and if the mast cells affected are in the head then the outcome might well be a streaming nose (chronic rhinitis).

Our biological structures are all as different as our finger prints, so the problems facing a practitioner specialising in allergic reactions (a clinical ecologist) are enormous and very complicated. A good analogy would be that of crossing a minefield. It was therefore only after a great deal of research and correlation of evidence that I decided to write this book, in the belief that with some guidance, millions of people all over the world, suffering from unnecessary allergy problems, might be able to negotiate the minefield with more safety than has previously been possible. There is no such thing as a diet for all men. We are all different and the old adage 'one man's meat is another man's poison' is never truer than when dealing with allergy reactions. Unless you are tested by a qualified practitioner (or learn to use the Davies method, of which more later), the only safe way of determining your allergy is by elimination.

METHODS OF TESTING FOR ALLERGY

The elimination method

This is long drawn out but effective. The only drawback is when there are multi-factorial problems; then it can appear almost impossible to determine the culprit. Not many people are allergic to lamb, pear or potato, so reduce your intake to these foods and Malvern water for five days. Then introduce one food from a different food family every five days, make sure no ill effects are experienced and continue adding a food at five day intervals.

During the initial period of five days you are almost certain to experience withdrawal symptoms. These vary to such a degree that it is very difficult to tell you what to expect, but the type of reaction you may get is as follows: headache, nausea, shaking, excessive perspiration, clamminess, aching in all joints, raised or lowered pulse rate, influenza type symptoms. The spectrum is wide and patients' comments range from 'I don't know why you made such a fuss, I hardly felt a thing' to 'You were quite right to warn me I might feel ill, for the first week or so I thought I was going to die'. Somewhere in that spectrum you will fall but it is impossible to determine where.

I remember saying to a lady, crippled with arthritis and in a wheel chair, 'You will probably have a very distressing time initially and it may go on for as long as three weeks. Try and bear with it, take pain killers if necessary for this period, once you are through the elimination period you are sure to feel better'. She rang three weeks later saying, 'I am out of my wheelchair, standing at the kitchen sink doing my washing up, where is all this pain I am going to have?'. I could only reply that she had either been very lucky or had been in so much pain previously that she did not notice the difference.

I also recall a man from Chepstow who had gout in both feet and ankles. I told him that he might experience quite a bit of discomfort for about ten days but that it should be easier after that. The poor man was on the 'phone to me for the next six weeks. The pain was indescribable and he was crawling to the loo on hands and knees, unable to put his feet to the floor. I begged him not to give up the diet and, full marks to him, he stuck it out; six weeks and three days later he put his shoes on, walked in comfort and, thank goodness, has had no recurrence of the problem since. *On average the withdrawal symptoms last five to ten days*.

The elimination diet of lamb, pear, potato and Malvern water should not be undertaken without first mentioning it to your doctor or under the supervision of a qualified practitioner, as the withdrawal symptoms can be quite severe. As I am trying to be more specific about what foods cause allergic reaction I do not propose to list the various methods of dieting that can be undertaken to detect food allergies. One pocket sized and cost effective booklet that gives excellent information on this subject is *Food Allergy* – a practical, easy guide. In

Appendix A I will give examples of the foods which are best to avoid and an elimination of toxins diet.

The 'scratch' test

This is a simple test in which an area of healthy skin is selected and cleansed with alcohol; then a tiny, painless scratch with a sterile needle is made. The scratch is so light that no blood is drawn; a drop of the allergen is placed on he skin and left for fifteen to thirty minutes, then wiped off. If the area becomes inflamed and irritable then a positive reaction is recorded. As many as one hundred tests can be done at one sitting.

The intradermal test

The intradermal test gets its name from the fact that the allergen is dissolved in liquid and injected into the skin. Another area of skin in close proximity to the first is then selected and clear liquid injected. It is then possible to compare the two for any redness or swelling which would indicate an allergic reaction. The intradermal ('into your skin') is often used because it gives a quicker reaction. The results may be read in from eight to fifteen minutes. Like the scratch test it is not painful but must be administered with care.

The patch test

An area of skin is cleansed with alcohol and a piece of gauze is dipped in the suspected allergen and then taped on to the skin. Checks can be made at regular intervals to observe any irritation or inflammation in the area. The gauze can be left for as long as three days to determine reaction. If the reaction were strong then it would be removed very quickly.

The eye test

If you are one of the many patients who react violently to

allergenic substances then the eye test may be used. The reactions to this test are milder although the readings are similar. A drop of the suspected allergen is placed in the corner of the eye and ten to fifteen minutes later the eye is carefully examined for any redness or irritation. It may cause the patient to sneeze violently, which would indicate an allergenic reaction. The symptoms usually wear off after thirty minutes to two hours.

The Davies test

The foods that are most commonly ingested are the ones tested first: tea, coffee, milk, flours, etc. These are placed, one at a time, under the tongue onto the sub-lingual and sub-mandibular salivary glands. These have an immediate nerve reflex contact with the pancreas. This nerve reflex can be likened to a fuse wire that acts as the 'breaker' between the nerve reflex and the very large group of muscles across the back, shoulder and upper arm – the latissimus dorsi, teres minor and triceps. Why test or challenge the pancreas? Because it controls our blood sugar levels and the whole of our digestive enzymatic processes. If you are not allergic to a particular food substance the muscle group will hold firm to the challenge. This is a pressure of three to five pounds exerted on the wrist across the stomach, but if you are allergic to a substance then the ability to hold that pressure becomes impossible. For want of a better description the nerve reflex fuses and the current to the main generator ceases. Non-scientific it may be, but simple, effective and painless it most certainly is.

It is important to make clear at this juncture that neither the sub-lingual test nor the use of muscle reflexes is an invention of mine. Dr. Guy Pfeiffer and Dr. Lawrence D. Dickey were responsible for refining the sub-lingual procedure around 1962. Their methodology is somewhat different to mine. Substances were placed under the tongue; the veins under the tongue are close to the surface and readily absorb traces of foods, drinks and drugs (it is for this reason that nitroglycerine and other drugs are placed under the tongue for immediate absorption). A careful procedure of taking the patient's pulse at rest and checking for any marked fluctuation in pulse rate when a food substance was placed under the tongue, and any alteration in pupil size, facial colour, respiration etc were carefully noted.

This method whilst very accurate and effective is by necessity time consuming. Dr. Richard Mackarness in his excellent book *Not all in the Mind* describes the techniques used and was certainly responsible for bringing to the attention of the medical profession and the public at large the possibility of an alternative method to determine food sensitivity. There must be a quicker way I thought to myself, and there was. I was invited to attend a seminar on Applied Kinesiology given by Brain H. Butler one of the best instructors of this technique in this country. It was after many months of studying these techniques that I became aware that more than one muscle group could be used to attain a positive response, I experimented for months before realising that it was the quick, easy and painless way I had been seeking. The evidence in this book is based on that procedure and perhaps in the future will help many practitioners to ascertain the aetiology of a patient's complaints.

THE PANCREAS

The Islets of Langerhans, part of the pancreas, contain about one million cells, glands of internal secretion generating a hormone known as insulin which is injected into the blood.

Insulin regulates the metabolism of carbohydrates and controls the blood sugar level. A deficiency in the production of insulin results in diabetes mellitus, commonly known as sugar diabetes, the condition in which the body is unable to use its blood sugar, which therefore builds up in the blood and has to be excreted by the kidneys. This state is called hyperglycaemia. By distinction the over activity of insulin through

13

dietary transgressions removes glucose from the blood by increased combustion and enlarges the store of glycogen at the expense of the glucose. This state is called hypo–glycaemia, and since the brain depends on a constant supply of glucose, sufferers can have a feeling of passing out, clamminess, sudden

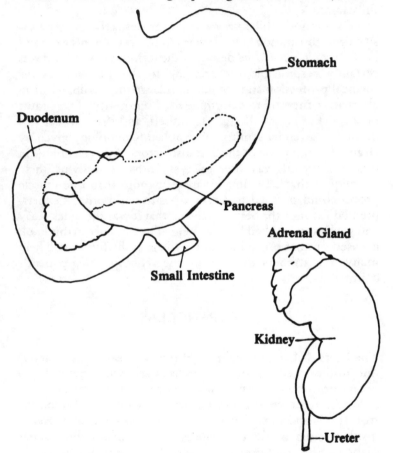

This diagram is not intended to be medically or anatomically accurate but to give you some idea of the organs that control your digestive system and therefore your health.

loss of energy, hunger, and in extreme cases epileptic seizures and sometimes collapse.

You will observe from this the importance of correct pancreatic function. It is our central computer and, like all computers, unless you feed the correct information in, then you will certainly not get the correct information out. I place paramount importance on pancreatic function, and all the tests carried out in my clinic are based on it. *We are what we eat.* The pancreas has the initial say on how well we are and the one way to undermine our health is to ignore the importance of the pancreas. It is the instigator of our whole digestive processes, and on the outcome of that enzymatic sensitivity rests the performance of our whole system.

I wish to stress at this point that the tests carried out in my clinic are performed by me. These tests are undertaken with the sole intention of making patients aware of their allergens and warning them of the consequences of continuing ingestion of these. If you suspect that you have a disorder of any kind, then consult your doctor or a qualified practitioner first. They will ascertain whether there is an organic failure or infection and treat accordingly. But, if you have been to your doctor and through the normal channels of investigation and you are told that there is nothing wrong with you, that all tests show a negative response, and that you must 'learn to live with it', then, and only then, consider the alternative I am suggesting to you.

REINTRODUCING ALLERGENIC SUBSTANCES

Once an allergenic substance has been removed from the diet, and the problem has gone completely, then you must take great care not to ingest this substance again for a period of three months. This will allow the metabolism to right itself and the self healing processes of nature to repair the damage. Before you introduce the substance back into your diet, check your pulse, sitting quietly. Introduce the incriminated substance as a single item, check the pulse twenty minutes later and thirty minutes after that check the pulse again. If there is a fluctuation up or down of more than twelve beats then there is evidence of a reaction. In some cases a dramatic reaction will leave you in no doubt. A lady recently returned six weeks after her first visit. Then, she had complained of an urticarial rash (hives), which produces, among other things, swelling of the hands. This time she was completely free from any symptoms. Over the festive season she had a small glass of sherry. On reporting back to me she said, 'I could hardly believe my eyes, within ten minutes both my hands were swollen, very red and painful.' This was an obvious reaction. Not all reactions are quite so obvious, but they are generally apparent.

Imagine your body as a pond (70% of our system is water). When you are in a toxic state the pond is very murky. If you threw a bucket of dirty water into the pond, you would not see a great deal of difference; the pond would appear more or less the same colour. However, once you have de-toxified the system and the pond is beautifully clear, then an egg cup of dirty water thrown in will produce a marked difference in the colour of the water, toxification taking place and creating far more disturbance than would previously have been noticeable. So please be warned; if you have discovered an allergenic substance and you really wish to re-introduce that substance, be prepared that it may have a deleterious effect on the system. If, however, you have re-tested and as far as you can detect there is no reaction, then introduce that substance every fourth day and make sure no reaction is experienced. By rotating in this way there is every chance of the adrenal glands being able to cope and produce enough adrenalin and cortisone to stabilise the situation.

My advice would always be, if you can cope without the substance, then you are far better off without it. Why put the system into an 'alarm' condition, strain the pancreas and kidneys and liver, when they are coping extremely well and you are healthy? The decision is yours alone.

16

IN CONCLUSION

As I said earlier, and really can not stress enough, do not treat the testing as a party game. Health is a very serious business, the most valuable asset you will ever be entrusted with, so take care of it, nurture it tenderly with love and care and you will be rewarded handsomely.

If you have one of the complaints we have discussed and you have consulted your doctor, the normal investigatory procedures have been carried out and no obvious physical or organic explanation can be given, then I suggest you consider the possibility of an allergen being the cause. I have referred to the fact earlier that all the testing carried out in my clinic is based on the reaction of that wonderful organ the pancreas. I have been saying for years that if we made sure the pancreas was functioning correctly then many of the chronic degenerative diseases prevalent in our society today would be eliminated. This is not a new idea but is becoming recognised slowly but surely as fact. In their wonderful book *Brain Allergies*, Dr W. Phillpott and Dwight Khalita, Ph.D. refer continually to the importance of pancreatic function and state that 'the pancreas is the first endocrine-exocrine organ influenced by contact with ingested foods and chemicals . . . It has the monumental task of buffering against reactions to any of these substances. Robert Forman, Ph. D., in his book *How to Control Your Allergies,* devotes a whole chapter to 'hypoglycaemia, allergy and the pancreas'. So you will see that the testing we have been carrying out is of great import and the conclusions we have drawn will I trust be of help and bring hope to many.

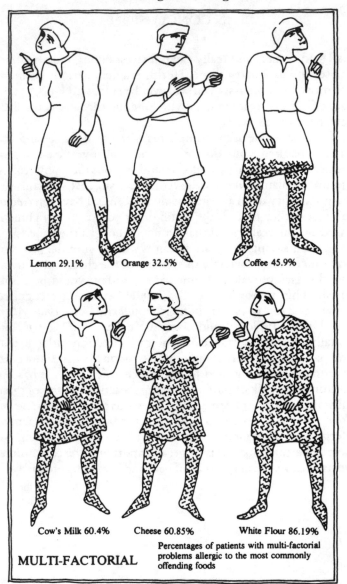

Lemon 29.1% Orange 32.5% Coffee 45.9%

Cow's Milk 60.4% Cheese 60.85% White Flour 86.19%

MULTI-FACTORIAL

Percentages of patients with multi-factorial problems allergic to the most commonly offending foods

ELIMINATION OF TOXINS DIET

Breakfast   Pure orange, grapefruit, pineapple, apple, blackcurrant or grape juice.★
Boiled, poached or scrambled egg. One slice wholewheat toast. Bowl of muesli with milk, cow, goat or sheep or soya.★

Lunch   Meat, cheese or fish with salad. Lettuce, chinese leaves, cress, beetroot, tomato, cucumber, peppers, celery, carrot etc.★ One slice of bread wholewheat. Fruit salad. Coffee. Tea. Caro. Pioneer, Barley cup. Postum. Chicory. Dandelion coffee.★

Tea or Snack   Glass of milk or pure fruit juice. Nuts. Seeds. Fruit.

Dinner   Soup (not thickened with flour). Lean meat: pork, ham, beef, lamb, turkey, pheasant, chicken, duck, rabbit.★ Potato, carrot, runner bean, broad bean, cabbage, cauliflower calibrese, sprouts, parsnip, swede, turnip, peas.★ Fresh fruit salad. Beverage or milk or fruit juice.★

★ Indicates a selection of the foods mentioned and nothing from a packet or tin.

CHAPTER 2

What foods are at fault?

I would stress at this point that I am not knocking any particular food or industry. The whole purpose of this book is to provide evidence of my findings over the years and, I hope, help many thousands of you suffering from a complaint that you have been told to live with. No one is infallible and I am the first to admit that failures are bound to occur, but the irrefutable fact is that by eliminating offending food substances you can obtain the most healing effect.

Only yesterday I had a young woman of 30 years of age return after six weeks eliminatory diet. On her first visit I stood at the top of the stairs and watched her ease her way gingerly up the stairs with the help of her husband. She asked me not to shake hands as they were too swollen and painful. She had been diagnosed by her doctor nine months earlier as having arthritis. She was quite tearful and naturally told me that as she was so young she did not want to 'live with it'. She complained of severe pain and swelling in the hands, knees and feet, total fatigue, chronic constipation (common in arthritics), premenstrual tension and menses very light, panic attacks and chronic anxiety and depression brought about by the sudden affliction of pain and deformative swellings. Her allergens followed an all too common pattern: MILK, WHITE FLOUR, ORANGE, RENNET, TOMATO, RHUBARB, GOOSEBERRY, CHEESE, BUTTER.

On her return yesterday she ran up the stairs looking radiant and said 'I don't really know why I am here, I feel absolutely wonderful – thank you'. On questioning I found that every one of her symptoms had disappeared, the swellings had gone, she had full mobility of all joints and no sign of the arthrosing condition at all.

I quote this case because it is so fresh in my mind and also because once again the two main culprits of disease were at fault – MILK and WHITE FLOUR.

MILK

Why milk? I wish I could give a straight forward answer to that, but it is so complicated and I have not had the chance to carry out enough detailed research to be specific. There are various schools of thought and it certainly is dangerous when dealing with infants not to ensure that their food intake is balanced and that a diet too high in protein is not used.

There is an awareness among lay men and women and the medical profession of the importance of cows milk in the aetiology of eczema, gastro intestinal disorders associated with the failure to thrive, and cot deaths. The alternatives are goats milk, sheep milk and soya milk. For adults this does not present too great a problem, but for infant feeding then professional advice should be sought.

The digestion of an infant is so delicate that great care must be taken when giving advice on the alternatives to cows milk. The BMA journal (22.9.79) stressed the importance of nutritional needs in alternative milks and recommended the use of *Prosobee* and *Velactin* for infant feeding. The article also condemned the use of *Plamil* but I believe the manufacturers have made concerted efforts in recent years to bring this product up to standard. For adult use there is now Soya *Granose* which is very palatable.

One point that must be raised here is the necessity of the Goat Society of Great Britain to get its house in order. As you will see on the appropriate diagram, cows milk is one of the leading suspects in many conditions, which necessitates the use of an alternative, a good wholesome nutritious alternative. In this part of the West Country we are extremely lucky: the Staple Lawns herd of goats, some 300 plus, are run in the same way as a dairy herd of cows. Strict codes of cleanliness are observed, the milk is checked frequently for bacteria, the milk proceeds direct from goat to tank via sterilised tubing, the temperature reduced rapidly and the milk passed straight into bags and sealed.

The feeding of the goats is very strictly supervised by Patrick and Barbara Chamberlain to their own formula. The success of their insistence on strict control of diet and cleanliness is apparent when one looks at this large herd and observes gleaming eyes, happy contented animals producing full quotas of first class milk, bacteria and mastitis free, summer and winter.

If all herds were run and fed on the same lines then I am sure the complaints I receive from patients of milk that tastes of the 'billy' and separates on de-frosting would not exist. A standard level of production should be reached and regulations governing the sale of goat milk must be tightened up, but the opportunity and the demand are there.

Several herds of sheep are now being run to produce milk. Although sheeps milk is more expensive it is certainly a delicious and nutritious alternative to cows milk. The following information will be of value to those of you who require an alternative and wish to make comparisons.

TABLE 1

Comparison between total solids, protein fat and ash, with some of the B complex vitamins in the milk of ewe, cow and goat

(Derived from Williams et al 1976)

	%EWE	COW	GOAT
Total Solids	18.2	12.1	11.2
Protein	4.3	3.4	2.9
Fat	8.4	3.5	3.9
Ash	0.83	0.75	0.79
Riboflavin mg/kg	4.3	2.2	1.4
Thiamin	1.2	0.5	0.5
Nicotinic acid	5.4	1.0	2.5
Pantothenic acid	5.3	3.4	3.6
Vitamin B6	0.7	0.5	0.6
Folic acid	0.054	0.06	0.06
Vitamin B12	0.0098	0.0035	0.0007
Biotin	0.05	0.025	0.04

TABLE II

Comparison between some specific constituents of the milks of the ewe, cow and goat. (N.I.R.D. 1981)

W.W.F.D.E.	=	Wield Wood Friesland Dairy Ewes.
N.I.R.D.S.	=	National Institute for Research in dairying Suffolks.
B.A. Goat	=	British Alpine Goat.
J.C.H.	=	Jersey Cow Herd.

	%W.W.F.D.E's	N.I.R.D.S.	B.A.Goats	J.C.H.
	19.8.81	11.8.81	10.7.81	25.6.81
Protein	5.98	5.85	2.63	3.81
Fat	5.79	6.45	2.75	5.10
Casein	4.94	5.19	2.31	3.26
Non Casein	1.04	0.66	0.32	0.55
Lactose	4.76	4.47	4.15	4.53
Somatic cellcount		310	392	706
915	x 10^3/ml.			

We have not included a table of the amino-acid composition of ewes milk, but the table in Williams et al (2) shows that the amino–acid concentrations in ewes and cows milk are broadly similar.

TABLE III

Comparison of some minerals in milk of ewe, goat and cow

		EWE	GOAT	COW
Ca.	g/litre	1.89–1.98	1.23	1.20 (3)
P.		1.43–1.57	0.90	0.92 (3)
Na.		0.41–0.53	0.35	0.48 (3)
Mg		0.17–0.19	0.13	0.22 (3)
Zn		5.16–5.54	3.29	3.50 (4)
Fe		0.66–0.86	0.50	0.50 (4)

Comparative figures for the ewe and goat are taken from Mathieu and Jaouen (1977) from a table in (i).

Sheep in Britain are free of brucella Ovis which is found in many other countries of the world. They are also free of brucella Melitensis, an organism often found in sheep and goats outside the United Kingdom and the cause of the well known Malta or undulant fever. Tuberculosis is very rare in sheep and the few recorded cases are usually in pet or orphan lambs kept in unsuitable environments.

Salmonellosis (a common cause of food poisoning) has been on the increase in recent years and outbreaks have occurred in humans from drinking unpasteurised milk and with increasing frequency from made up foods. As a disease it is far less prevalent among sheep than bovines, particularly calves. The common species of salmonella, Dublin and Typhimurium usually reported in cattle are seldom found in sheep; of those reported occasionally in sheep, salmonella Newport appears to be the most usual.

The transmission of salmonella amongst beasts is from animal to animal, the young calf, because of the pattern of trade, being an example. Young lambs are, however, not sold in markets and there is no trade in this class of stock. The other source, in poultry particularly, is by infected material of animal origin included in feeding stuffs. This is less of a danger in sheep due to the fact that such feeding stuffs are unlikely to form part of the compound rations of a dairy ewe; also, almost their entire lactation period is spent out at grass.

It would, however, appear desirable that any milk obtained from an unknown source should be pasteurised, not boiled. Boiling may well destroy the very benefits to be found in sheeps milk.

To pasteurise small quantities

Put the milk in a double saucepan or fireproof jug in a saucepan of water and either heat the milk to 62.9°C (145.22°F) and hold it at that temperature for half an hour or heat the milk to 71.6°C (160.88°F) for 15 seconds. Cool as rapidly as possible in a closed vessel.

A big test for the Milk Marketing Board

Milk, the lovely 'pinta' that we are encouraged to ingest and trained from very young children to accept and regard as a necessary staple food *can* be one of the most harmful. The Ministry of Agriculture will no doubt attempt to discredit any suggestion that milk could be harmful; after all it is a vast money-making product with vested interests running to millions of pounds. But one cannot get away from the facts:

1. *The only milk God clearly intended us to ingest is the milk of our Mothers*, and then only for a limited period before we are weaned from the breast to ingest solids. The same thing applies to the cow. If left to its own devices the cow will feed the calf until it is old enough to ingest grass; then the cow dries

up and replenishes its own body with the minerals and vitamins it requires.

2. *Is it a coincidence that the country that has the highest consumption of milk products – Finland – has the highest male mortality rate from coronary thrombosis in the world?* The figure drops in countries with less consumption down to near zero in third world countries, many of whose inhabitants are allergic to milk anyway.

3. *How many suffer from milk allergy?* The chart on page 95 will indicate how many of my patients are allergic to milk. Figures in the United States indicate that 58% of those of ethnic extraction and 18% of whites are allergic to milk. I have indicated previously the types of conditions that lactose insufficiency can trigger and they are numerous, but as the result of the correlation of evidence over a five year period the following are the main conditions associated with milk allergy:

> PSORIASIS   ECZEMA   COLITIS
> DIVERTICULITIS   ASTHMA   ANGINA

The latter complaint is not only a distressing but frightening condition, and in my experience not one of the patients I have found allergic to milk have had problems afterwards. The pain invariably goes within five days, any attendant Hypertension (High Blood Pressure) reduces within three weeks and the remark most commonly heard is that 'I feel better than I have done for many years'.

The Ministry of Agriculture, *not the Department of Health* is responsible for the continued encouragement of milk consumption in schools. The natural outcome of over-subsidisation and the ensuing butter and cheese mountains and milk lake is the need to try and sell these products to the nation as being 'good' for us when in fact any dietician worth their salt would hesitate before recommending the daily ingestion of large quantities of milk, butter and cheese.

The saturated fats contained in these products are medically proven to be contributory factors to heart disease and my tests have certainly borne this out to the full. Milk has become identified with coronary heart disease, which causes 150,000 deaths a year in this country alone. Both milk fats and skimmed milk appear to be atherogenic, contributing to the build up of plaque in artery walls.

Apart from the commercial considerations, and they are vast, the danger is also with us of too much penicillin in milk. The failure rate in England and Wales of 1.5 per cent is the highest in Europe, ten times as bad as some other countries. The risk here is that too many people are running the risk of building up resistance to antibiotics through regular exposure to small amounts of penicillin in their milk.

Adult man is the only animal on this planet to remain dependent on infant food. We have been so brain washed and stomach washed by milk that it is not easy to be weaned from it. I refer to milk in general, not just the milk of the cow. We have become dependent on milk to put in our tea and coffee and over our cereals, utilising an animal baby food for our trained palate. I am convinced that if we left animal milk products in general to the infants of the animal kingdom, for whom they are intended, then we as humans would all benefit from a health aspect.

Needless to say this would be totally unacceptable economically. *Here's Health* July/August 1983: 'At present there is an EEC surplus of some 1.4 million tonnes of skimmed milk powder'. That is the tip of the iceberg and I do not expect any responsible body to take note of my cry in the wilderness, or of the many more powerful lobbies presenting evidence of the ill effect of continuous milk ingestion, but you, the reader, can take action. You can if you wish eliminate milk from your diet completely, read the labels on tins and packets avidly and make absolutely sure you do not have milk in any of its disguises without knowing it. Less obvious forms include skimmed milk, lactose, lactic acid, whey, casein and caseinates. There follows a list of some of the foods that contain milk. This is not a complete list and manufacturers change the contents of their products continuously, but it should give you a guide.

FOODS CONTAINING MILK

The under-mentioned products can, and frequently do, contain milk in one form or another.

Baking powder
Biscuits
Baker's bread
Bavarian cream
Blancmange
Boiled salad dressings
Bologna
Butter
Buttermilk
Butter sauces
Cakes
Chocolates
Chocolate or cocoa drinks or mixtures
Cream
Creamed foods
Cream sauces
Cheeses
Curds
Custards
Doughnuts
Eggs scrambled and escalloped dishes
Rarebits
Salad dressings
Sherbets
Souffles

Foods prepared au gratin, foods fried in butter (fish, poultry, beef, pork,), flour mixtures, fritters, gravies
Hash
Hard sauces
Ice creams
Malted Milk
Ovaltine
Meat loaf
Cooked sausages
Milk chocolate
Milk in all forms
Omelets
Oleomargarines
Pie crust made with milk products
Popcorn
Popovers
Prepared food mixes for biscuits, cakes, doughnuts, muffins, pancake, pie crust, waffles and puddings
Soups
Sweets
Junket

WHITE FLOUR

The following is a list of the proposed new Food Regulations governing the use of additives in flour products – bread, biscuits, cakes, etc. If anyone can offer me a logical and sensible answer to the question, why are these additives necessary, and whom do they benefit? then I will be willing to climb down from my soap box, tail between legs and skulk off admitting that I have been scaremongering all along. But until that time, and I do not think that will ever occur, I shall shout as loudly as I can with every means at my disposal that because of regulations such as these the nation as a whole is being slowly poisoned and bludgeoned in to the rash of chronic degenerative diseases prevalent in our society today. Look at the list and ask yourself why? Why should a natural product like wheat, already tampered with by the application of mould-killing sprays, be denatured to such an extent that it needs FIFTY-TWO additives made available for bakers to use to make a consumable product?' The fifty-two are

E 150 Caramel
E 170 Calcium carbonate
E 220 Sulphur dioxide
E 221 Sodium sulphite
E 222 Sodium hydrogen sulphite
E 223 Sodium metabisulphates
E 224 Potassium metabisulphite
E 226 Calcium sulphite
E 227 Calcium hydrogen sulphite
E 260 Acetic acid
E 262 Sodium hydrogen diacetate
E 270 Lactic acid
E 280 Propionic acid
E 281 Sodium propionate
E 282 Calcium propionate
E 283 Potassium propionate
E 290 Carbon dioxide
E 300 Ascorbic acid

E 322 Lecithins
E 330 Citric acid
E 333 triCalcium citrate
E 336 monoPotassium L-tartrate
E 341 Calcium tetrahydrogen diorthophosphate
E 450 diSodium dihydrogen diphosphate
E 460 Alpha-cellulose
E 465 Ethylmethylcellulose
E 466 Carboxylmethylcellulose, sodium salt
E 471 Mono- and di-glycerides of fatty acids
E 472(b) Lactic acid esters of mono- and di-glycerides of fatty acids
E 472(c) Citric acid esters of mono- and di-glycerides of fatty acids
E 472(e) Mono- and diacetyltartaric acid esters of mono- and di-glycerides of fatty acids
E 481 Sodium stearoyl-2-lactylate
E 482 Calcium stearoyl-2-lactylate
E 483 Stearyl tartrate
(500) Sodium hydrogen carbonate
(510) Ammonium chloride
(516) Calcium sulphate
(541) Sodium aluminium phosphate, acidic
(641) D-Glucono-1, 5-lactone
(920) L-cysteine hydrochloride
(924) Potassium bromate
(925) Chlorine
(926) Chlorine dioxide
(927) Azodicarbonamide
Ammonium dihydrogen orthophosphate
diAmmonium hydrogen orthophosphate
Ammonium sulphate
Amylases
Proteinases
Nitrogen
Benzoyl peroxide

Wheat before milling is treated with benzoyl chloride as a bleaching agent. Traces of this remain after the process and are a prime cause of allergy or intolerance.

You would have needed to be an industrial chemist to understand most of these constituents, until now. At long last there is a guide which enables all of us concerned with nutrition to enlighten ourselves and those we are entrusted to help.*

With the aid of this reference book you will be able to see what most of these items are and most important of all how 'nutritious' they are. If you consider that is too high a price to pay for this valuable information then a free booklet is available from the Ministry of Agriculture entitled *Look at the Label*. This is invaluable advice, but if the items on the label are indecipherable then what good are they? Look at the label please, it is so important to realise what it is you are ingesting. Many of these products are often not what they are purported to be, and certainly do not resemble a natural product.

You will see on page 95 that white flour is one of the two most predominant allergens, along with milk. The reasons for this are quite logical – the two most common substances ingested day after day by the great majority of the public are milk and white flour. If cigarettes warrant a warning that smoking can damage your health then white flour should have a skull and crossbones on the packet and the axiom 'The whiter the bread, the quicker you're dead'.

I must stress again that I am not knocking a particular industry, purely a product that does irreparable harm. Wholemeal flour is easy enough to produce, longer to rise and therefore more time consuming, but a much more acceptable and nutritious substance. Proponents of the white loaf will say it is equivalent if not better than the wholemeal loaf because it has 'enriched' vitamins and minerals put back into it. I am always reminded of a story Abraham Hoffer tells in his book *Orthomolecular Nutrition* when this subject is aired; it goes something like this. You are walking along a street and a mugger pulls a gun on you and orders you to strip naked. The thief takes your clothes and valuables. Noticing your shiver-

---

* *E for Additives, the Complete E Number Guide* by Maurice Hanssen (Thorsons, £2.95)

ing embarrassment he returns your underclothes and gives you fifty pence to catch the bus home. Do you feel enriched?

One young lady who did not feel enriched was brought to see me two years ago. I shall call her Wendy to protect her anonymity. Wendy was eighteen years of age and was accompanied by her mother. Just as well, for I could not get one word out of Wendy herself. She sat in the chair looking very pale and totally disinterested in everything I was saying. She obviously was not well and had no intention of contributing information that would help me discover the cause of her condition. I did not really want the mother to answer for Wendy, but that was the only avenue left open to me.

G.H.D.: What is wrong with your daughter please, she does not look well.

Mother: No, she is not well and yet she is not ill as such, from the age of thirteen she slowly retracted into her shell, not intersted in going out, tired all the time, in fact a zombie.

G.H.D.: Has she been like this continuously or is it just moodiness?

Mother: No, I don't think it is moods, just total withdrawal from the world.

G.H.D.: I will ask you some questions to see if any of these symptoms sound like Wendy's.

I then proceeded with the questionnaire. There certainly appeared to be nothing organically wrong, purely a pancreatic maladaption problem; in simple terminology Wendy was being 'poisoned'.

I tested her and found her to be allergic to white flour and sugar. The possibility of withdrawal symptoms was very strong, so I advised the mother to watch Wendy carefully for at least seven days. In fact there was no need for concern, as she came through the first week with no great difficulty and after that became better by the day. Three weeks later she went for a holiday in Spain and, a few months later, applied for and secured a job in Austria as a groom. I am glad to say that she has kept in touch over the last year or so and is still enjoying life to the full.

Her mother was quite angry when she realised what had caused her daughter's decline and she lobbied her member of parliament and wrote to the papers on the issue, but of course it made no impact. Only when the government, with all its power, bans the use of additives and preservatives in white flour, as the French government has done, will we as a nation benefit. Look how healthy this nation was at the end of the second world war. The amount of artificial ingredients in our food then was at a minimum, and don't tell me that the bread was not more edible then. I can remember my mother being absolutely furious after she had sent me to the local bakers for a loaf and I returned with loaf minus crust. It really was delicious.

The only way that things are going to change dramatically is for you to refuse your child the plastic loaf and insist that wholewheat flour is used. Then perhaps the multi conglomerates will alter their 'recipes', the educational authorities will realise why their classes are full of naughty children and in domestic science classes they will actually learn to cook with wholewheat flour. Then the producers will go back to the good old days and allow us to make a choice. Sounds good, doesn't it? In an ideal world of course we should not be exposed to all these dangerous chemicals, of which no one knows the long term effects, but this is not an ideal world. It is one where the awareness of the public is being aroused and more wholewheat bread and flour is in demand, but beware, they are ahead of you. As soon as it became apparent that wholewheat bread was in demand then production went up. But have you ever looked at a wholemeal loaf, not at the loaf itself, but at the packet? In large letters it will proclaim 100% STONEGROUND WHOLEMEAL FLOUR. Absolutely true, but less easy to see are the small letters which say PERMITTED ADDITIVES. It is these which can harm. They are fewer than in a white loaf but are there none the less.

Hidden enemies

With the advent of new regulations governing additives in food, next year should see some clarification of contents. At present the manufacturers think of all sorts of wording to disguise the use of white flour; hopefully this will not be the case in 1986, although I have no doubt that manufacturers will find some loophole to allow them to continue.

When buying wholewheat flour you need 100% for bread making, 81% or 85% for pastry making. Use plain, not self raising and baking powder which does not contain white flour (in the UK, Boots and Sainsbury's fulfil this condition). You can of course make your own with two parts bicarbonate of soda to one part cream of tartar, and you can use rice flour to help the free flowing of stored amounts. If you wish to make a sponge then sieve the flour until all the coarse grain is removed, using the coarse grain for an apple crumble; then the fine flour should make an acceptable sponge. Adding one teaspoon of bicarbonate to every eight ounces of flour will certainly make it rise.

DO REMEMBER – PACKET BREADS ARE OUT!

HYPERACTIVITY

This is a wide subject and one that arouses great passion because children are involved. Whether one accepts that food could be a contributory factor, or not, any practitioner should at least consider the possibility of foods creating a metabolic disturbance and if there is no improvement in the condition then proceed with further exploratory examination. I have often had nursing mothers come with their 3 month or 6 month old child complaining that the child cries continually or has obvious colic. The first question is of course 'are you still breast feeding?'. Invariably the answer is yes. I then test the mother and find out her allergens; within days of the elimination of these the child is settling down and sleeping properly.

What are the first signs of hyperactivity? The inability to sit still for any length of time, flitting from one occupation to another rapidly, fiddling, twitching, foot tapping, bottom wriggling, bad temper, irrational temper tantrum at the slightest provocation, sleepless nights. One mother a few years ago came with her son of six and they had not had one night's sleep in that six years. Hyperactive children often find it difficult to smile.

In infants the reaction is most likely to be one to milk, wheat or eggs ingested by the mother and passed on to the child. As the child gets older and more commercial foods are used then the problem obviously becomes more involved, but it would be fair to say that if the youngster is kept off packaged foods and fed on whole grain, fresh vegetables and fruit, meat, fish and substitute milk, then the chance of finding the offending food is enhanced. Different children, like their adult counterparts, react to different substances, so it is impossible to be specific, but as a general guide the elimination of food colourings also helps to produce a favourable response.

Hyperactive behaviour in children due to food sensitivity was first described by Doctor Theron Randolph in 1947. Since then many investigators such as Dr. A. H. Rowe, Dr. Frederick Speer, Dr. Stephen Lockey, and Dr. Ben Feingold have elaborated and explained these relationships. I have attempted to absorb and use the suggestions made by these pioneers and there is no doubt in my mind that there is often a link between hyperactivity and ingestants.

Are you a teacher? Perhaps you recognise that disruptive child in your class who drives you to distraction because he will not concentrate, cannot sit still, twiddles with his pencil or pens, twists his hair through his fingers continuously, is slow to respond and finds it difficult to concentrate. You could do that child a great service. You could suggest to the parents that hyperkinesis is not unusual, it carries no stigma, but is recognised in many cases as being related to allergy. With your guidance and understanding of the problem the parents will no doubt seek help and another child destined for nature's scrap heap will lead a normal active life.

If you as a reader of this book know of similar cases to the one I am about to mention, then do at least suggest that allergy could be the problem. You will not always be listened to, but even if you only sow the seeds then there is at least a possibility that at some time they will respond and you will have saved a child from years of misery.

Bernt was an eight year old who from birth had been difficult, never sleeping properly, crying a lot, being restless and bad tempered to the point of uncontrollable rages where everything in sight was thrown; in short, an impossible child. The parents naturally wanted their child to be normal. They approached their general practitioner who prescribed a drug to quieten him down. This worked initially to ease the situation but did not cure. The next step was a psychologist and further drugs were used, year after year, but no real relief was obtained and Bernt carried on being a horrible child. He never asked for or gave affection to his parents in any way, until in the end his behaviour was so intolerable that they firmly believed he was possessed by the devil and agreed to Bernt being admitted to a special psychiatric unit in Southern Germany.

Five days prior to this committal his Aunt asked me if I thought it was worthwhile bringing the boy to me as a last resort. How often I hear that term, the last resort. How I wish and sincerely hope that, like some, the majority of my patients will say I came to see you first as a preventive measure. I naturally informed the Aunt that at the stage Bernt was at, anything was worth a go. She rang the parents right away and they set off from Southern Germany on a five hour drive to North Germany. They brought the 'horror' in to my surgery, scowling and cursing under his breath: no way was he going to co-operate. I asked the parents to sit down and not worry

36

about Bernt nosing around the room, investigating everything in sight. I asked them to understand that it was not the boy's fault, that he was not possessed by the devil but was being overactivated by what could be an allergic reaction.

Naturally they looked at me with disbelief; how could a food or foods create such a destructive reaction? I then related several cases of boys and girls affected in a similar way and how they had responded well. Slowly I saw a change in the parents attitude and a glimmer of interest from Bernt. He eventually agreed to be tested and I found him allergic to five substances, including colourings. I warned the parents that we might not see any reaction for days and that our time was terribly limited. At least Bernt agreed to co-operate, as he did not want to go to the 'special school'.

Five days later, at eight in the morning, I had a phone call from the mother. Bernt had gone into the parent's bedroom, sat on the edge of the bed, put his arms around his mother and said 'meine liebe Mutti', my dear Mother, the very first sign ever of affection. The breakthrough – the small miracle we had all prayed for had happened.

It was not all plain sailing, Bernt still had his problems when he ingested toxic substances intentionally or unintentionally. On one occasion he sneaked off to his bedroom and his mother followed him. Bernt, unaware that he was being watched, starting revolving on the spot, slowly at first, then faster and faster until he was very hot, red faced and panting. He stamped his foot, cursed under his breath and said 'Why can't I get angry and upset, it used to work before. I must have some cake that will make me angry'. So you see he was not completely cured, something was still activating his system enough to make him want to be angry. But I am pleased to tell you that he is now much more rational and is not afraid of showing affection to his parents or relations.

I mentioned earlier that it is not easy to adapt to these procedures. It does not concern just the child, it would be most unfair for every other member of the family to go on eating normally. It will make for healthier cuisine for everyone, and a healthier climate for the hyperactive child when all temptation is removed.

Needless to say it is not just additives and colourings that are at fault but it is a good starting point to see how the child reacts to the elimination of these. If you can read then you can eliminate artifical colour, artifical flavourings, and preservatives from your shopping basket. At first it will be very time consuming reading every label on every item you pick up, but take a notebook with you and make a note of foods that are safe, whether you intend purchasing them that day or not. Remember to check them though, manufacturers do alter the ingredients without any warning.

There are many additives. Here is a list of a few, and once you recognise these names it will help in recognising the chemical names of others at a later date.

E NUMBER	NAME	USES
	Artificial colours	Many
	Artificial preservatives	Many
E 320 BHA	Butylated hydroxyanisol	Delays or retards the development in food of rancidity or flavour deterioration due to oxidation
E 321 BAT	Butylated hydroxytuolene	Antioxidant for food oils and fats
E 282	Calcium propionate	As a preservative and mould inhibitor
E 210	Benzoic acid	Antibacterial and anti-fungal
E 414	Gum arabic	Retardation of sugar crystallization, thickener, emulsifier, stabilizer and glazing agent
E 621	Monosodium glutamate	Flavour enhancer, stimulates the taste buds
E 405	Propyline glycol alginate	Emulsifier or stabiliser or

		thickener
E 211	Sodium benzoate	Preservative, anti-bacterial, antifungal
E 251	Sodium Nitrite	Preservative, Curing salt
	Brominated vegetable oils	
	Disodium benzoate	
	Saccharin	
	Sodium acid pyro-phosphate	

The easiest way of course is to avoid all foods contaminated with artificial flavourings and preservatives; keep to the whole foods, the natural foods. If possible grow your own without the use of artifical fertilisers and pesticidal sprays. If you cannot grow them, contact one of the agencies in the back of this book and they will put you in touch with local outlets. Those of us connected with clinical ecology started as a very small family, but it is growing every day and there should be help available in your area if not in your town or village.

To end this chapter I include an article written by a patient of mine. Jenny has started and runs successfully a support group in Weston-Super-Mare. The case-history is typical of so many youngsters. It could help you.

FOOD FOR THOUGHT:

by Jenny Davies*

How many times have we heard a mother say 'I can't think what's got into him to-day?', but I wonder how many of you realise the truth that lies behind those few words. I don't doubt that after reading this article you will look at that statement,

* Published as a leaflet by The National Association of Nursery and Family Care.

the children and their diet in a very different light.

Imagine my joy in finding myself pregnant. After a good pregnancy and a short labour my little Holly was born. She was perfect, beautiful. I cried.

I had already decided I was going to breast feed and all went well; she fed well and I enjoyed it. Unfortunately the Nursing Home insisted that you were not disturbed at night and so baby was given a bottle. Those bottles were the beginning of our problems. By the fourth day, Holly already had a reputation with the night staff as being difficult. When we came home things improved a little as she had very few complement feeds. Those of you who have breast fed will know the pressure that is put on you by well-meaning people that if baby cries, it's because she's hungry and you haven't got enough milk, so top her up. Not knowing anything better I did so and things got worse. By four months I gave up, convinced I was a failure. (My second baby, may I point out, I fed for 9 months and didn't listen to anyone.)

Holly was put on the bottle and things got worse. I was like a zombie. She slept for about an hour during the day and four at night, interrupted with feeds and crying. My husband was marvellous and took a lot of the load, but I still felt a wreck. We all went to the doctor, who viewed us with mild amusement and prescribed Phenergan for Holly, which was supposed to knock her out. It did the exact opposite – we now know that this was due to the colouring in medicine. By 10 months she was walking, talking a little; she did not sleep at all during the day and was constantly moaning. The nights were awful – I was in and out of bed all night. As a matter of interest, not all hyperkinetic children have a sleep problem.

I tried the doctor again and he referred us to a Consultant Paediatrician whose only statement was that Holly was a dynamic baby and why should she sleep. We left with me in tears. I thought 'Damn them all – I will get through it alone'.

By the time Holly was 14 months, I was feeling really down. I couldn't seem to cope with the house, and our marriage was put under a tremendous strain. There never seemed to be a moment to be together; our love life was hopeless with Holly always crying or, when she was older, standing beside the bed; you never knew when she would walk in on you. I became neurotic about noise when she was asleep: avoiding floor boards which made a noise, never pulling the flush, even disconnecting the door bell.

I felt I needed an outlet so, with a friend, we started a Pram and Toddlers Group. I enjoyed it very much, but it did very little for Holly – she ran around like a whirlwind.

I have always thought that an only child was wrong – it didn't seem fair – but at that time the thought of another baby made me feel ill. When Holly was 3 we decided to take the plunge and try for another, hoping that a baby would help us all. Holly loved everyone else's babies so much. When we told her we were going to have a baby she was thrilled. However, when he arrived the story changed. She was so jealous, I couldn't believe it. I couldn't change him without her going and doing something naughty. Every time I started to feed she would want something and it was always 'It's not fair, you always have Peter'. One friend suggested I gave up breast feeding, but I didn't see why Peter should be deprived. Life was hell and I hated her for all the unhappiness she brought me, all the things I couldn't do, places we didn't dare go. I could feel the atmosphere when I went to friends – only one or two gave me total support and would even invite me when Holly was really awful. I would never want to relive those first two months with the new baby again.

I was at breaking point – something had to be done. The doctor had given me Valium for her to try and get some peace but it made her wild; she lay on the Hall floor and screamed 'Don't touch me'.

I was getting to the point where I was afraid to smack Holly or even get cross in case I couldn't stop. On one occasion, I shut her in her room and rang my husband to come home, I was so afraid that if she went on I would really hurt her.

A friend put forward a suggestion. She had been to a Private Clinic to be tested for food allergies to try and help her with

41

her depression. She had been helped so much that she thought it might be worth taking Holly to see if she was allergic to any food.

We went as a family to the Clinic to meet Mr. Davies. To my amazement he was not at all surprised at our story or at Holly's behaviour. I told him how much worse her behaviour became after she had been to a birthday party.

He was very sweet with Holly and asked her to sit on his couch. He said he was going to see if different foods made her strong or wobbly. He put a tiny bit of each different food under her tongue and then with her right elbow tightly against her side, he gently pushed her hand toward her chest and asked her to resist, if she could. The first test was for tea and Holly was able to resist his pressure, thus showing she was not allergic. Then came coffee. Mr. Davies asked Holly to resist but as he applied pressure and she tried to resist, her arm went wobbly. She turned to me and the expression of fear and wonder on her face as to why she had no strength, told me this was no fix. With a sip of water between each test, Mr. Davies continued.

At the end, I was bemused. She had shown she was allergic to coffee, chocolate, citrus, white flour, white sugar, cows milk, cheese, colouring and preservatives, including flavourings. Peas and bananas came under colourings as they produce their own natural colourings. What was I going to feed her on? Mr. Davies warned us she might well suffer from withdrawal symptoms for the first week. In fact things went really well. I decided we would all go on Holly's diet. I emptied my cupboards of any foods she could not have and gave them all away. I was determined this had to be the answer.

The first week *was* like an answer to a prayer. Within two days she began to sleep thirteen or fourteen hours a night and I would find her asleep on the floor in the lounge. This excess of sleep lasted about five days. After this, as now, she slept for about ten hours. The jealousy eased towards the baby and her general attitude toward everyone changed. I began to enjoy seeing her first thing in the morning – a feeling I had not experienced for a long time. I also had to *learn* to love her.

The diet itself was a little tricky until I had worked out some substitutes. We have 100% wholewheat for bread and 85% for cakes and pastry. I make my own baking powder from rice flour, bicarbonate of soda, and cream of tartar. We have pure cane sugar instead of white, goat's milk instead of cow's, animal rennet-free cheese and mazola oil instead of margarine for cooking. I have become a compulsive label reader and if it doesn't say what's in it, I don't buy it.

Everything was going really well and people who knew Holly remarked on the change; but we were not out of the woods yet. After several weeks of what seemed like heaven, Holly began to get difficult at bedtime and sometimes during the day. Then one day it clicked, as she came and told me for the third time that morning, that she had cleaned her teeth. I rushed upstairs and looked at the toothpaste tube. It was nearly empty. I couldn't believe it – she was eating the toothpaste! It never occurred to me that the stripe in the new tube would have any effect on her, but she felt it and began to crave it. I changed the toothpaste and things returned to normal.

After something like twelve months of good days and nights we began to have problems. Her teacher also noticed the change and wondered if it was the excitement of the approaching Christmas Nativity, but I could see all the old signs returning as well! Constant uncontrolled laughter, silly faces, wild eyes and the old faithfuls, bad nights and the constant movement. I rang Mr. Davies who suggested a retest.

Mr. Davies greeted Holly like an old friend, smiled at me and said 'Yes, I can see it'. I told him an average day's menu and he started the tests.

He hadn't gone far when goat's milk showed as an allergy. Both of us were surprised – where did we go from here? Soya milk was the answer. She was also allergic this time to the white of egg but this didn't pose too much of a problem as I just give her two yolks. So we plod on again once more with a pleasant child. However we have to take care not to give Holly

43

any one food or drink in excess, as it is possible for her to build up an allergy to it.

An interesting point I think is that food allergies seem to run in families. If there is a child with a behaviour problem – look at the family: does anyone have asthma, eczema, migraine, hay-fever, depression, ear infections or even a skin or intestinal problem? The child's behaviour could be due to food allergies, although not in all cases.

I have now started a local group for mothers of children who have been tested by Mr. Davies. Not all the children are first babies or only children. We give support and swap ideas for recipes.

I hope that some of you, having read this article, will be able to see that something could be done to help a child, or perhaps a family you know. Let there be a happy end to the sad story of hyperkinetic children.

CHAPTER 3

Rheumatism and Arthritis

INTRODUCTION

Arthritis is one of the most common systemic physical diseases in advanced countries. There are an estimated eight million sufferers in Britain alone. There are two main types of arthritis, rheumatoid and osteoarthritis; rheumatoid arthritis can begin at any age, but usually is found earlier in a person's life than osteo or degenerative arthritis, which is more characteristic of old people.

So called traumatic arthritis may develop into either rheumatoid or osteoarthritis, and mixed arthritis with features of both rheumatoid and osteo is common. It is possible for any joint, or joints to be involved in rheumatoid or osteoarthritis but the joints of the hands are particularly vulnerable. In osteoarthritis it is most common to see the terminal joints of the fingers affected. In rheumatoid arthritis the second finger joints and knuckles are usually involved. It affects all of us in different ways. In some cases it takes months and sometimes years for it to become clearly a case of arthritis at all. An ache here or a twinge there is put down either to growing up or growing old. The joints slowly become more affected until swelling or severe pain occurs and then of course the correct diagnosis is made. In other cases it has literally come on overnight. There may have been odd muscular aches over the years but nothing serious; then one night the patient goes to bed as normal and, either in the night or in the morning, wakes with severe pain and aching 'hot' muscles (myalgia), unable to move properly.

The outcome is the same – arthritis.

In his book, *Allergies – Your Hidden Enemy*, Theron

Randolph devotes a whole chapter to arthritis and the association between this condition and food substances and chemical susceptibility. The first definitive work was published by Doctor Michael Zeller in 1949 and titled *Rheumatoid Arthritis – Food Allergy as a Factor*. These men were the pioneers of clinical ecology and its use in the relief of debilitating diseases.

Since the 1920s medical practitioners have been recording individual maladaptive reactions to foods and chemicals observed as emerging during controlled systematic test exposures.

The tests I have carried out as indicated by the graph provide conclusive evidence that the pancreas, as the instigatory endocrine-exocrine organ, gives us the key to relieving many of the debilitating conditions prevalent in society today.

Arthritis, in all its guises – and they are numerous, is an inflammatory condition.

One of the most important functions of the pancreas is to supply proteolytic enzymes (enzymes from the pancreas that aid in the digestion of proteins to amino acids) which act as regulatory mechanism over inflammatory reactions in the body. Several substances in the human body are capable of producing inflammatory reactions. Among these are tissue hormones known as KININS. Kinin reactions are usually the most frequent, the most severe and the most painful. Inappropriate release of these hormones is caused by inflammatory substances (foods, chemicals, etc.) to which a person may be allergic.

Without going into great detail about how this reaction affects the liver, kidneys and other organs, I hope it will be apparent that elimination of allergenic substances, rotation of diet and avoidance of chemicals in various forms will provide the body with enough natural energy to commence the recuperative procedures necessary for recovery.

I would like to close these introductory remarks by quoting a paragraph from a book called *Brain Allergies – The Psycho-nutrient Connection* by William H. Philpott M.D. and Dwight Kalita Ph. D.

The 'hard way' to discover truth need not be the only one. We must always keep in mind that the greatest enemy of any science or any discovery of truth is a closed mind. Accordingly, we should seek the courage to ask impertinent questions which will shake our complacency and challenge our minds to look deeper into the farthest reaches of the great mystery of the human body. Then and only then will we be able 'to accept truth at face value'.

WHAT CAN BE DONE ABOUT ARTHRITIS?

In the following pages I give methods which, if followed properly will ameliorate and in many cases cure rheumatoid and osteo arthritis, the dreadful crippling diseases from which, on latest estimates, 7 million people in this country are suffering. You will no doubt notice similarities to books by various other authors, who have said that this way or that way is the only true way to cure the condition. But I make no such claim. We are each as different as our finger prints, and obviously my method will not suit everyone. I have had patients crippled by the condition who, when told the regimen necessary to effect relief, have considered it too high a price to pay, and have continued eating their sticky buns, cream and jam, or continued drinking alcohol at the expense of their health. No one can help you unless you wish to be helped.

Over the years many hundreds of patients who have had the intelligence to carry out the instructions have gained tremendous relief. A publican, for instance, had knees so swollen and painful that he had had to abandon his true love, golf, and was then threatened with having to give up the public house. Within six weeks the swellings had receded, he no longer had thoughts of giving up his livelihood, and now he is back on the golf course and thoroughly enjoying life. Another example is of a young girl of seventeen who had been slowed to a snail's

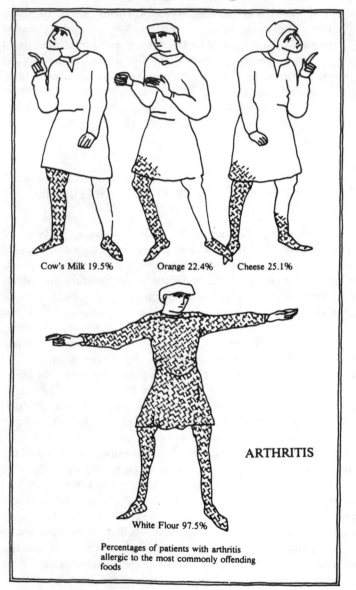

Cow's Milk 19.5%   Orange 22.4%   Cheese 25.1%

ARTHRITIS

White Flour 97.5%

Percentages of patients with arthritis
allergic to the most commonly offending
foods

pace by the pains and swellings that racked her body. Within six weeks, on her return visit, she was able to run up the stairs, smiling all over her face. The swellings had gone and so had the pain. She was able to resume her duties with the St. Johns Ambulance service with, I am sure, thanks to her superior officer who had paid her consultation fees.

The point I would like to make now is probably the most important one of all. I have found that unless you are tested for food allergies there is a distinct possibility that the recommendations I make in this chapter may not suit you at all. Remember, we really are all individuals. One man's meat is literally another man's poison. I had one elderly lady of 73, severely crippled with arthritis, who, after six weeks on the restrictive mode of eating, had made great strides. The swellings had reduced considerably but she was still getting a lot of back pain. On more detailed testing it was found she was reacting to prunes, which were eaten on most days. On removing these from her diet she was able to report in three weeks that the pains in her back had gone.

The point I am trying to bring home very positively is that although I am sure that the method of eating, and the foods recommended, will be beneficial to many thousands of arthritic sufferers, if it does not work for you then do not be disheartened and think that the end of the road has been reached. You may be one of those people who need to consult a Clinical Ecologist and determine whether you have a food sensitivity problem.

One young lady of 23 was severely affected by arthritis and in a great deal of pain. On testing she was found to be clear on egg and cheese, so after three weeks on a *week one diet,* (see page 56) and now free of pain, she introduced eggs and immediately had a reaction. She waited until she was free of pain and introduced cheese, with the same reaction. You may well ask, what was the point of testing her then? The answer is fairly straightforward. Because her system was so toxic on the first test, only the predominant allergies were apparent. Having cleared these from her system, the lesser allergens were able to come to the fore and have a severe effect. On rechecking her foods I was able to confirm the reaction to egg and cheese and since then she has made remarkable progress and is living a pain-free life.

The well-known Naturopath Harry Benjamin, N.D. once wrote

> By the very nature of the case, such quick and definite results as those which follow the treatment for simple rheumatism cannot be expected (in treating arthritis). Natural treatment holds out the only hope of cure – or even partial cure – that exists in the world today. Orthodox medical treatment, by means of injection or otherwise, is worse than useless where real cure is concerned. The sufferer from arthritis, more so than any other, can afford no longer to tamper with their diet if a cure – or even partial cure is wished for.

The mention of drugs is one that we must dwell on for a moment. Most people have heard of drugs such as Butazolidine and Opren, once considered safe, which have now been withdrawn. What of other drugs which we take for granted? Is the common aspirin entirely safe? The short answer must be no. All drugs have some side effect. Some of these side effects are most debilitating, worse than the condition being treated. I could go into a lengthy discussion on the side effects of drugs, particularly those for arthritic conditions, but I will not bore you with these. I just point out to you very forcibly that any drug taken over a reasonable length of time will most certainly have a severely deleterious effect on the tissues and organs of the body, with the chance of irreparable damage being done. I would suggest, if you are taking a drug prescribed by your Doctor, that you check it out. There is an excellent book by Peter Parish called *Medicines, a Guide for Everybody*. Then, if you are about to embark on the programme I am suggesting you should adopt the following procedure. After three weeks you should have found that the awful deep gnawing, aching pain and any swellings have reduced. Then I would suggest that you reduce your intake of the drug slowly and surely. BUT, consult your doctor if you are taking steroids. If you are on four tablets a day reduce to three, if you are on one a day, reduce to one every other day. By this method you should determine when you are pain free, and that point is where you remove the drug completely, I hope for ever more.

Very many patients have come to me and said, 'I had terrible swellings and the pain was unbearable, so the Doctor suggested I saw a Rheumatologist and he recommended gold injections'. I look at these patients and ask, 'How long was it before the symptoms returned?' Invariably the answer is 'two or three years, but then the symptoms returned and became as bad as ever'. It is a sad fact that gold injections, though they do have a miraculously curative effect at first, convincing the patient that the condition is cured, do eventually allow the 'old enemy' to return with a vengeance. Then what is to be done? Increasing the dosage is not the answer. Sadly, I have to warn you that if you have had gold injections the proposals I will be making for the majority of those suffering from arthritis will not necessarily be applicable to you. The blood platelets are altered to such a degree that the chances of a natural recovery are much reduced. It has worked for some, and I am therefore recommending that it would certainly be worth your while to try it, but be prepared for the sad fact that it might not.

I certainly would not wish to pretend that the road you are about to embark on is an easy one. It will be pretty hard for a number of reasons. One particular difficulty is in your social life. It becomes extremely difficult to accept cocktail or dinner party invitations unless the host is a particularly good friend and is willing to cater for you. It would be true to say that it is at times like these that one discovers who one's real friends are. Do not be put off by feeling the 'odd one out'. You have a genuine illness. Unless someone has suffered it himself it is very difficult to comprehend in others. Be open and honest and tell them that you can not have certain things because they have a very painful after-effect, and you have suffered long

51

enough not to invite the 'old enemy' back again. Eating out could also be difficult, but if you choose a straightforward meal like steak and salad, then you should have no problems. You will not worry because you will know full well that any deviation from the straight and narrow will have painful repercussions, but your family and friends will worry for you. It is up to you to convince them that you are very happy with what you have, and resist the temptations put your way by the most well meaning people. They are not the ones who are going to suffer – you are!

You will have to re-think all your eating habits, and your food buying habits too. You will have to use a positive approach – 'I will defeat this dreadful painful disease' – then you will be on the road to a normal healthy way of life, free from pain. Gradually you will be able to introduce 'forbidden' foods, once the disease is under control, but should there be a reaction then of course that particular food must be banished for ever. Your health will depend upon your honesty with yourself.

What can you expect once you start your new way of eating? One thing is almost certain: you will suffer withdrawal symptoms. This means that by withdrawing from foods that have been part of your every day eating habits, a withdrawal reaction is almost certain to come. A correlation can be made with the alcoholic being withdrawn from his tipple, or a drug addict being removed from his 'fix'.

What will happen? The withdrawal symptoms vary in length of time and severity. They cover a spectrum from 'I don't know what you made all the fuss about' to 'I wish you had written that seventy feet high. If someone had dug a hole and pushed me in during that first fortnight, I would have said thank you'.

WITHDRAWAL SYMPTOMS

The typical withdrawal symptoms are a feeling of having influenza, aching of all parts of the body, high temperature, severe headaches, palpitations, pains in parts of the body that have not been affected before and, in some cases, the feeling that one is going to die. Thankfully, that has never occurred with any of my patients and as far as I am aware, neither has it occurred elsewhere. It is a very tough time to get through, make no mistake about it, but if you grit your teeth and say 'I will beat this dreadful disease', then you will make it. The length of time the withdrawal symptoms take again varies, from a week to six weeks. Generally speaking the worst of the symptoms are over within the first fortnight.

The following is a list of foods that must be excluded. Put it up in your kitchen commit it to memory, never forget it. You will note that raw foods are best for the first week or so, but if you can not face that, then cook very gently, just enough to soften and use the juices to drink with the meal or to make a soup.

TOXINS – POISONS – NEVER TO BE TOUCHED

Prepared and processed foods; pre-packaged desserts; tinned foods (soups, meats, vegetables, fish, poultry); cakes; sweets; ice cream; certain meats (pork, ham, bacon, veal); packetted cereals; all flour products (spaghetti, pasta, etc.); refined rice products; pizza; coffee; tea; soft drinks; jams; sugar; artificial sweeteners; imitation dairy products; wine; beer; spirits; any food tampered with by man

The obvious conclusion on reading this list is to think 'What can I eat?'. Plenty: you can eat fresh meat, fish, fresh fruit, fresh vegetables, natural cheeses, eggs, nuts and natural sweeteners. If you stick to a diet based on these foods then you are likely to remain pain-free. If you choose to ignore this advice then you have only yourself to blame.

Shelf space in your pantry will become less of a necessity, that is reserved for foods designed to have a long life and preserved accordingly. Refrigerator and deep freeze space will be required for organic 'live' foods such as lettuce, brassicas, beans, peas, carrots, swede, turnip, onion and fresh organic fruits. If it is home produced so much the better. YOU NEED NOT SUFFER ARTHRITIS.

The real causes of arthritis are

1.   *The inability of the digestive system to tolerate certain foods and drinks (allergy)*

2.   *A scarcity of the nutrients required by the body to function correctly.*

3.   *An overabundance of chemical additives used in the processing of foods which our bodies do not need, and can not cope with (toxicity).*

At the risk of repeating what so many authors have already said, I would like to remind you once again of the tribe in West Pakistan called the Hunzas, one of whom I met at a conference in London recently. The Hunzas live to well over 100 years old. Common illnesses rare; heart attacks, cancer and child-hood illness uncommon. Mental illness is very rare and so is divorce. This perhaps sounds too good to be true but the answer can be found, at least partly, in the Hunza diet. It is largely made up of fresh vegetables (uncontaminated by modern fertilisers), whole grains, fruits and berries, (fresh and sun dried), butter, cheeses and milk which may be fresh or soured. I do not encourage the drinking of sour milk, but just think what happens to our own milk. It is pasteurized or homogenised. This entails putting it under high pressure and elevated temperature, which changes the raw protein, making it less nutritional and destroying the enzyme phosphotase which is essential for the utilisation of calcium and phosphorous. It also destroys most of the B and C vitamins.

54

So you see, you do not have to take bigger, better or stronger pills. It is simpler and in a way worse than that! You are going to give up some of the foods and drinks you have been used to all your life. For some this will be a bitter pill indeed, but you can cure your arthritis if you want to.

The following is a list of seventeen common food additives. Over the next few years I am sure they will officially be proved to be harmful to the human system.

1. BHA. 2. BHT. 3. Benzoate of Soda. 4. Caramel. 5. Carrageenan. 6. Dipotassium phosphate. 7. Disodium dihydrogen phosphotase. 8. Food colourings. 9. Monosodium Glutamate. 10. Oxygen Interceptor. 11. Polysorbate 60. 12. Polysorbate 80. 13. Sodium nitrate. 14. Sodium nitrite. 15. Sodium silico aluminate. 16. Sorbitan. 17. Sulphur dioxide.

Now think carefully about the situation. These seventeen additives are used in food production today. The list is quite an eye opener but imagine it trebled, plus, for just one product. White flour has up to 52 permissible additives and chemicals. There are more than 3,000 permissible additives and we are the guinea pigs at the end of that line. It is only in recent years that we have begun to reap the harvest that was sown when government bowed to the greedy manufacturers and allowed additives to be used.

Do you not consider that we should take time to think carefully why we need so many replacement kidneys, heart transplants and organ replacements? Why there are so many diabetics? Why there are so many hyperactive children and why there is so much juvenile delinquency? Why there is such a high crime rate? Figures are available for all these categories, and in recent years many reports published by eminent men have pointed a finger at food as the one trigger factor.

YOUR DIET

The following diet is based on that in Giraud W. Campbell's book, *A Doctor's Proven New Home Cure for Arthritis*, published in the UK by Thorsons Publishers. Reading this book seven years ago first made me aware that the dreadful crippling effects of arthritis could in fact be linked with the ingestion of certain foods. I have altered and added to some of the things Campbell advocates, in the light of my own practical experience. However, it remains a basic, sensible, no frills diet.

The diet I advocate will I hope eliminate the worst trouble makers and help to make your life more tolerable. You are going to embark on a body wracking journey that is to rid your body of all the toxins and start you on the road to health and pain free living. Start now with this positive thought: I NEED NOT SUFFER ARTHRITIS.

Day One

Breakfast	–	None	Drink only water, at least 8
Lunch	–	None	glasses during this day. (Do not repeat this water day. If
Dinner	–	None	you are still in pain after seven days then repeat the first week again but begin on Day Two.)

Day Two

Breakfast	–	Unsweetened fruit juice. Banana (ripe), pear or apple.
Lunch	–	Fresh chicken. Mixed green salad, oil and vinegar dressing. Bowl of fruit in season.
Dinner	–	Vegetable salad (raw celery, carrots, cabbage, etc.). Raw fruit salad (shredded peeled apples, figs, grapes, bananas, etc., but no citrus).

56

Take one tablespoon of cod liver oil or ten capsules at night, with milk or a fruit drink, at least two hours after food.

Day Three

Breakfast   –   Blended raw fruits. 8 fl oz untreated or gold top milk.

Lunch   –   Fresh fish, lightly cooked.
Raw cauliflower or other raw vegetables.
4 RNA/DNA tablets. 1 tablespoon blackstrap molasses or 4 capsules.

Dinner   –   Fresh (or Kosher) beef lightly sauteed with onions. Mixed green salad. Melon or other fruit in season. 8 fl oz untreated milk.
Cod liver oil capsules with fruit juice or milk at least two hours after food.

Day Four

Breakfast   –   Prunes or prune juice. 8 fl oz untreated milk.

Lunch   –   Lamb chop or roast lamb.
Mixed green salad.
8 fl oz untreated milk. 4 RNA/DNA tablets. 1 tablespoon blackstrap molasses or 4 capsules.

Dinner   –   Grilled Dover sole, plaice etc.
Mixed green salad. Half avocado pear. Fruit in season. 8 fl oz untreated milk. One tablespoon or 10 capsules of cod liver oil at night with milk or fruit drink, at least two hours after food.

Day Five

Breadfast   –   Melon, or other fruit in season. 8 fl oz untreated milk.

Lunch   –   Half avocado, mixed green salad. 8 fl oz untreated milk. 4 RNA/DNA tablets. 1 tablespoon blackstrap molasses or 4 capsules.

Dinner   –   Fresh beef. Mixed green salad. Fruit in season. 8 fl oz untreated milk. One tablespoon or 10 capsules cod liver oil at night with milk or fruit drink, at least two hours after food.

Day Six

Breakfast   –   Unsweetened grape or prune juice. Bubble and squeak. 8 fl oz untreated milk.

Lunch   –   Shrimp salad. Melon, or fruit in season. 8 fl oz untreated milk. 4 RNA/DNA tablets. 1 tablespoon blackstrap molasses or 4 capsules.

Dinner   –   Large chef's salad, including raw peas, string beans, and other uncooked vegetables and greens. Plums or fruit in season. 8 fl oz untreated milk. One tablespoon or 10 capsules cod liver oil at night with milk or fruit drink, a least two hours after food.

Day Seven

Breakfast   –   Sliced bananas. 8 fl oz untreated milk.

Lunch   –   Lightly broiled fillet of sole. Carrots, watercress. Grapes. 8 fl oz untreated milk. 4 RNA/DNA tablets.
1 tablespoon blackstrap molasses or 4 capsules.

Dinner   –   Lightly sauteed kidneys or meat of your choice. Raw vegetables chopped in blender.
Melon or other fruit in season.
One tablespoonful or 10 capsules of cod liver oil at night with milk or fruit drink, at least two hours after food.

NOTE   Raspberry and other berry fruits may be used, but not strawberry or gooseberry. No rhubarb. No smoked fish or meat.

Special instructions for all seven days

1. Drink only when thirsty, and then only raw fresh fruit juice or juice of raw fresh vegetables, untreated milk, or water.
2. Substitute foods according to taste, or those seasonally available. But please remember never from a packet or tin.
3. Continue with the seven day regimen until pain, heat and swelling are gone.
4. When the pain, heat and swelling have gone then add *one food at a time* from the allowable list attached. Make sure that the food you introduce does not produce any adverse reaction.
5. Make sure you shop in advance for the items you require. Remember the Scout motto and 'Be prepared'.

FOODS THAT MUST NEVER BE EATEN AGAIN

Please excuse me for repeating these items but it is so necessary for you to appreciate how important this is. Because of the practical problems of managing without flour and patients' reluctance to do so, I try to introduce whole wheat flour back into the diet after three months. Naturally everything must be alright, no pain, swelling or stiffness of joints. But I must stress that the degree of success with this introduction is very finely balanced and is most certainly fifty/fifty at present. Fifty per cent report that they are very relieved to have bread again with no apparent problems. The other fifty per cent tell a much different story. Within hours, or in some cases days, the pain and swellings have returned, or they are stiffening up again. So please proceed with great caution.

Strictly speaking you should avoid the following altogether – *today and tomorrow*. The more you adhere to the strict regimen of the diet the more healthy tomorrows you will have.

The following are to be excluded for a pain-free life

1. At least for six weeks exclude all flour products, whether made from whole wheat, white flour, rye flour, buckwheat, millet or soya flour.

2. Tea, coffee, cocoa, alcoholic drinks (spirits, beer, wine), still and fizzy soft drinks. Drink fresh fruit juices only, avoiding lemon or orange initially.

3. Sugar or artificial sweeteners, and products such as sweets and ice cream.

4. Jams and marmalades. Home made jam with fructose is allowed at a later stage.

5. Tinned or processed foods. Foods manufactured, prepared or semi-prepared by man, including breakfast cereals.

6. Frozen fruit, unless organically grown and frozen yourself.

Do not cheat, for you only cheat yourself.

Basic list of recommended foods

1. FISH: Cod, crab, dover sole, halibut, hake, herring, huss, lemon sole, lobster, mackerel, plaice, rock salmon, salmon (not smoked), trout, tuna, etc.

2. FOWL: Chicken (free range if possible), duck, goose, pheasant, turkey.

3. FRUIT: Apple (peeled), banana, blackberry, cherry, currants, date, fig, grape, loganberry, melon, nectarine, peach, pear, plum, raspberry.

4. MEAT: Beef (roasts of all kinds), steak (all kinds), shank, rib, minced beef, flank, stewing beef, ox tail, mince (no preservatives).

Pork (roasts of all kinds), chops (all kinds), pigs trotters, spare rib, sausages (home made).
Lamb (roasts of all kinds), chops, shank and shoulder.
Organ meats occasionally.

5. NUTS: Almond, brazil, cashew, chestnut, coconut, hazel, peanut, pecan, walnut.

6. SEEDS: Pumpkin, sesame, sunflower.

7. VEGETABLES: Asparagus, broad beans, broccoli, brown rice, brussel sprouts, calabrese, carrots, cauliflower, chive, corn on the cob, courgettes, cress, cucumber, egg plant, endive, garlic, horseradish, kale, kohl rabi, leek, lentils, lettuce, marrow, mushroom, onion, parsley, parsnips, peas, red cabbage, runner beans, salsify, savoy cabbage, shallots, split peas, spring onions, swede, turnips, watercress. Treat tomato, beetroot and radish with caution, avoiding all together in the initial stages.

If you can obtain free range eggs, or cheese straight from the farm, then please do so.

Vegetarian cheese, is also a very good cheese.

Points to remember

1. Balance your menu as well as possible between protein, fat and carbohydrate.

2. Cook foods as little as possible; use the juice you cook them in.

3. Always eat raw vegetables or fruit at every meal.

4. Do not use the juices from the meats for gravy, as any impurities will be concentrated in these.

CHAPTER 4

Migraine

One in five families throughout the world has an inherited migraine problem. In an average street of fifty houses, ten people will be suffering the dreadful debilitating effects of a migraine. If you are one of the unlucky ones you have my deepest sympathy for, of all the allergic responses to food or fluid, this to my mind is the worst.

WHAT IS MIGRAINE?

Visual disturbance

A narrowing of vision, flashing lights, rainbow effects, jagged streaks of light in the corner of one or both eyes, twitching of eye muscles, double vision, where normally clear cut images become blurred and split in two.

Nausea

The awful churning and lurching feeling in the stomach, knowing that at any moment you could be sick, and on many occasions actually vomiting. In many cases this does ease the terrible pain and the symptoms begin to recede. This is due to the toxins which have built up in the system being released and the adrenal glands slowly recovering.

Pain

The pain of a migraine has to be experienced to be fully understood. It is far greater than any ordinary headache. I have heard it described as 'the brain being pulled in opposite directions by two very strong teams of horses'. The pain is usually so intense that the only relief possible is to retire to a darkened room, lie down and apply a cold compress to the head. I have known fully grown men and women scream and bang their heads against the wall with the pain. If you know any one who suffers in this way then please tell them that they *do not have to live with it*.

WHAT CAN BE DONE ABOUT MIGRAINE?

When migraine is mentioned one naturally thinks of someone suffering a frightful head-ache. I have had many dozens of patients with very bad stomach pains which had been diagnosed as colitis or diverticulitis, and in some cases Crohns disease, and on testing were found to conform to the migraine pattern. They were in fact suffering from a gut migraine. So if you have been to see a specialist and it has been confirmed that nothing organically wrong can be determined, and that you must learn to live with the migraine – eliminate the foods I suggest later and see if the problem resolves itself after ten days.

It is not a new idea to suggest that food is connected with migraine – the disability has been known since the time of Hippocrates – and it is not new to suggest that certain foods can 'trigger' an attack. Mrs Jones cut out chocolate and coffee from her diet and never had another migraine. Lucky Mrs Jones, for she quickly found the answer, but there are thousands of others who suspect a food such as cheese or chocolate, or even both, and eliminate them only to find the headaches persist. In these persistent cases where the 'trigger' foods or drinks have been impossible to determine, it is invariably a

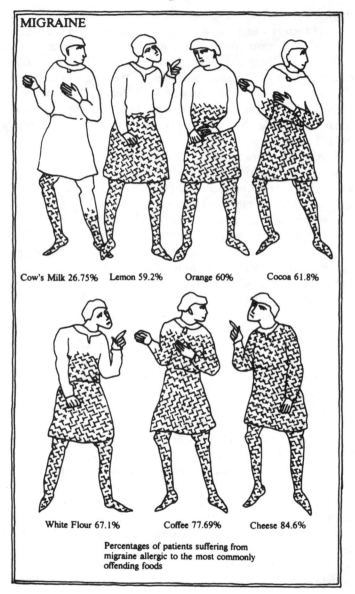

MIGRAINE

Cow's Milk 26.75%   Lemon 59.2%   Orange 60%   Cocoa 61.8%

White Flour 67.1%   Coffee 77.69%   Cheese 84.6%

Percentages of patients suffering from
migraine allergic to the most commonly
offending foods

65

multi-factorial problem. So where do you start?

Eight weeks ago a lawyer came to see me and told me that he had seen numerous specialists in Harley Street and had attended the Migraine Centre in London, all to no avail. He had suffered a migraine headache of varying intensity every day of his life. For twenty-seven years he had not had a pain-free day. I cannot imagine having a headache every day: it makes one realise how the human body will adapt and cope for quite long periods.

I told this unfortunate man that if he followed the advice I gave, there would be a very good chance of relief. He gave me a very old fashioned look and said, 'Yes, and I shall believe in ghosts, I need not tell you I am very sceptical'. I agreed that his scepticism was quite natural after all this time, and told him that I heard stories like his every day of my life but that I hoped I could change things. I then went on to explain what happens when toxic substances are ingested. How one moves through the three stages of the General Adaptation Syndrome. These are as follows. *Stage One*: perhaps as a small child you are fed egg, milk or cheese and either have a bilious attack or stomach ache. Mother quite naturally assumes that you are off colour but does not consider that this could be an allergic rejection and continues to feed you these foods. You then move on to *Stage Two* where the body does in fact learn to live with them – the adaptation phase. But slowly, yet inexorably, the pendulum swings towards *Stage Three*, the exhaustion stage. Then comes the migraine attack.

Each time you ingest a toxin, two things happen. One is that the adrenal glands that sit on top of the kidneys, where they should be the size of healthy walnuts, have to pump to produce adrenalin and cortisone in order to build up antibodies and keep us on an even keel. Slowly but surely, with the continuous ingestion of toxins, the adrenal glands atrophy (shrink) until they are the size of little hazelnuts, producing less and less adrenalin and cortisone, until eventually the toxins take over and a reaction occurs. At the same time the anti-bodies that are produced attach themselves to mast cells in the body. In the part of the body where the mast cells are weakest the allergy will manifest itself. Thus, if it is in the nose – hay fever, in the head – migraine. While the antibodies are attaching themselves to the mast cells you will keep on an even keel. Then the circuit is completed and two things happen simultaneously: the adrenal glands become exhausted and the mast cells 'flip' and shrug off the antibodies. The system is flooded with toxins and a reaction occurs.

Although looking slightly bemused the poor chap agreed that it seemed to make sense, and said it was the first time he had really understood what was happening. Then I went on to explain the test and how I would use his arm as a diagnostic tool to ascertain his allergens. While he had looked sceptical before, now he looked thoroughly disbelieving. I am sure he thought that this was just too simple a method to find out why he had suffered such agony for the best part of his life. I found that he was indeed a 'classic' case, manifesting the reactions that have become so familiar to me. They form a pattern which you may find helpful to characterize as the *4C syndrome*:

COFFEE   CITRUS   CHEESE   CHOCOLATE

Six weeks later our lawyer friend returned to shake me vigorously by the hand and inform me that he now believed in ghosts. I need not tell you that he was very pleased and full of joie de vivre. He asked me why others do not use this method, adding that in spite of his long period of suffering and the various drugs which had been tried on him, he had had no relief whatsoever. 'Yet', he said, 'I come to you, you "push my arm over", tell me to keep free of certain foods and for the first time I can remember for donkeys years I wake up free of pain. Mind you, you were quite right. My God I suffered for the first three days, the works: pain, nausea, flashing lights. It started to tail off on the third day and on the fourth morning I woke up without a headache.'

I do not know why others do not use the method. It is not easy for the layman. Applied kinesiology, of which this method is an aspect, has to be learned over many years and the biological and neurological functions of the body need to be properly understood. But there is no reason on earth why a doctor or practitioner could not apply himself and in a comparatively short time use the method successfully. I have been referred to by doctors and specialists in my area as a 'witch doctor'. This is a classic example of the lack of interest in alternative medicine amongst the orthodox medicine profession and shows ignorance of the true potential of clinical ecology and applied kinesiology.

All I really want you to do is to appreciate that over the years patterns have emerged that clearly implicate certain foods and drinks as prime suspects. The graphs on the following pages will show quite clearly which foods and drinks these are. If you eliminate all of them and find relief, then introduce one at a time until you find your 'trigger' foods. Then you will have made headway.

The chief things you must be prepared for when you eliminate these 'prime suspects' are the withdrawal symptoms. They can be quite severe. I have heard the following question so often from patients: 'You mean I am going to get withdrawal symptoms and feel ill just because I eliminate a few foods from my diet?'. Yes, you will have to accept the strong probability of severe withdrawal symptoms. The degree varies considerably, from those who say that they hardly felt anything at all to those who said they had to lock themselves away for three days. We are individuals and each one of us reacts differently, but on average it takes approximately five days before the worst of the reaction is over, and for those with slower metabolisms, anything up to three weeks. So do be prepared for at least forty eight hours of discomfort which could be quite severe.

THE 4C SYNDROME PLUS

As I have said previously, migraine is generally a multi-factorial problem and therefore difficult to ameliorate unless one is fairly sure of the contributory 'trigger' foods. The 4C Syndrome often has attendant allergens. These are inclined to be more peripheral and at a later stage such foods may be reintroduced. Having said that, they must be treated very seriously initially until the toxins have been eliminated completely and a stable situation realised for at least three months. It is then reasonable to assume that these peripheral allergens can be introduced in small amounts, once a week initially, to observe any unfavourable reaction. If all is clear on these initial introductions I would suggest that the foods be eaten twice a week with comparative safety as long as the amounts eaten are kept fairly small.

What are these foods?

Tomato, Onion, Garlic, Leek, Chives, Apple skin (peel your apples), Cider, Cider vinegar, Apple juice, Marmite*, Spices*, Nuts*, Legumes*, White Flour.

When you are allergic to Citrus it is not as easy as it may at first sound because it means that anything with citric acid in it must be treated with extreme caution. Alcoholic drinks become a problem for many, and an awful lot of my patients suffering from migraine state that they have given up alcohol altogether because they have found this a 'trigger'. While I am not recommending the ingestion of alcohol, it is not necessary in most cases to ban it altogether. 'Mixers' create a problem because most of them contain citric acid. You should certainly not drink red wine, port or sherry, but a good quality white wine may be tried to ascertain if there is any adverse reaction.

Numerous foods contain citric acid, so check every packet and tin you buy: dangers are lurking in the most unexpected places. I remember a lady from Newbury who had suffered from migraine headaches for most of her life and who had a

---

* The items marked with a star are those that have been found to be lesser incriminatory foods whereas Tomato and Onion are frequently implicated.

headache of varying degree every day. After testing it was clear that she had the classic 4C syndrome plus and I warned her that the withdrawal symptoms might be quite severe. On her return six weeks later she confirmed that this was the case and that she was left with a 'muzzy' head. The second test was carried out and we found the culprits.

I did not see this lady for approximately three months, when she came with her daughter, suffering from asthma. Quite naturally I asked her how she was and she was clearly delighted that she was feeling on top of the world. I asked if she had experienced another migraine attack and she said yes, one. I asked if that had been an error or a test to see if a food could be introduced. No, it was an error. She had been invited to a dinner party by a friend and explained that she would love to go but had to be careful what foods she ate because the slightest slip-up gave her a headache. Her friend assured her that the meal would be prepared in such a way that she could eat everything. So, feeling very happy that her friend understood, off she went. Hors d'oeuvres – fine; main course – fine; dessert – suspicions entered her mind, for although it was apple she felt sure she could taste LEMON. She whispered to her hostess, who assured her that all was well, so she continued with her dessert. A few minutes later she asked her hostess again and oh dear! – she had used lemon to prevent the apples from going black.

She left the party and drove home, I believe a ten to fifteen minute drive, parked her car in the garage, locked the garage door and walked to the front door. That is all she remembers for she was 'out'. Her husband had to help her to bed and she was poorly for forty eight hours afterwards.

ELIMINATING THE 4C SYNDROME

Coffee   Fairly simple to eliminate as it is not hidden in many other foods. I am continuously asked is decaffeinated coffee permissible. The answer is emphatically NO. Coffee is coffee is coffee. OUT!

Chocolate   Again fairly simple to eliminate as it is obvious. If there is no allergy to milk then Carob powder and Kalibu chocolate can be used as a substitute.

Cheese   I have found with testing many thousand migraine sufferers that the 'trigger' factor in cheese is in fact the rennet. So, providing you obtain animal rennet-free cheese, then all should be well.

Citrus   The most difficult one of all to eliminate. It is in so many foods and drinks. But providing you are constantly on the alert then you should manage very well. After all, anything is worth the effort if you are migraine free. Avoid the following: lemon, orange, lime, pineapple, tomato, citric acid, citrates, grapefruit.

Onion   If you do find these are a problem then I would suggest you eliminate the whole onion family initially: onion, leek, garlic, chives, shallot. There are many instances of patients being able to have one or other of this group with no reaction at all. Some have stated they can have them raw and not cooked, others that they can have them cooked but not raw, so you see it is a very individual thing and must be worked out by you.

CONCLUSION

There really are no hard and fast rules where allergens are concerned. Certainly, unless you are tested you must proceed with caution, but if you adopt the following procedure then there is a very good chance you can eliminate migraine forever.

Eliminate the foods and drinks stated in the 4C Syndrome: coffee, cheese, chocolate, citrus and citrates. The withdrawal symptoms are usually felt after the first twenty four hours of avoidance, so if you can time it to coincide with a week end off then so much the better. Remember they can be quite severe, so be prepared. You may be one of the lucky ones and not feel a thing. Make absolutely sure that none of the peripheral foods are clouding the issue: tomato, onion, apple skin, cider, cider vinegar. If in doubt then eliminate these and add them one at a time at a later date.

Rotate your foods as much as possible so that the chances of building up a reaction to a food is avoided. If you like apricots, peaches, plums, gooseberries, pears, or any other fruit, then do not have too many at one time, and certainly attempt to rotate them every three to four days. In her excellent book called *Good Food to fight Migraine,* Hilda Cherry Hills lists numerous recipes which I am sure you will find helpful.

CHAPTER 5

Asthma, Eczema, Psoriasis and Allied Skin Conditions

In the previous chapters I have been able to pinpoint certain foods as being contributory to a specific condition. They repeat themselves hundreds of times over, so that it is comparitively simple to correlate the symptom and the effect, and pinpoint the implicated ingestants.

With skin conditions and asthma this is not the case. I would go as far as unequivocally to implicate milk and white flour in skin conditions and say that they are a good base for anyone to work from. Sadly it is never quite as easy as that. I only wish it were, for then the number of people able to help themselves would mutiply rapidly.

I had a letter this morning from a lady with eczema. She has been very good with her diet, but has not been too successful in the first few months. There was an improvement, no doubt, but not as much as she or I had hoped. I asked her to send me a diet list for seven days of every item she ingested. When I received the list it was obvious that she ingested far too much coffee, at least 3 – 4 cups in the morning and the same in the afternoon. I asked her to eliminate coffee for at least three weeks, which she did and the eczema has at last started to diminish, although the skin is still very dry. This dryness is usually a vitamin and mineral deficiency and I shall advise her accordingly.

With all these conditions there is a correlation between reaction and the ingestion of additives and preservatives in food and drink. So when dealing with these symptoms I would advise you to look at the label carefully and if at all suspicious, do not touch.

Which foods are predominant? MILK, WHITE FLOUR, CITRUS, TOMATO, ORANGE, FLAVOURED CRISPS, ALCOHOL, APPLE PEEL, COFFEE, ONION, MIXED NUTS, MIXED HERBS, EGG, SUGAR, SALT, PORK, HAM, BACON, VEAL, MARMITE.

Now I realise as well as you that it would take months to eliminate these items one at a time, and with a list as long as this one the chances of cross permutation are high and could run into many thousands. There is no easy solution and there never will be where allergens are concerned. It is hard work, patience and alertness that count. Patience is probably the highest on the list for the frustrations are many and it is relative. If you have only a small patch of eczema, or you wheeze occasionally then you are not going to devote a lot of time and energy to eliminate a minor irritation.

It is a different story if you are smothered in eczema or psoriasis, or you find it difficult to walk one hundred yards without the aid of an inhaler. Then you would want to devote time to the cause and eliminate it if possible. So start by eliminating all MILK and WHITE FLOUR products. Keep the diet as simple as possible for a week. Do not starve yourself, follow the elimination of toxins diet. At the end of a week you should have noticed a considerable change for the better, if that is the case then introduce another product every three days and watch for reactions.

If, for instance, you find after a week that your wheezing has abated and your breathing is much easier then introduce a food every three days. If you find that on the introduction of onion, for example, you have breathing problems or your catarrhal condition worsens, then eliminate the whole onion family – ONION, GARLIC, LEEKS, CHIVES, SHALLOT, SPRING ONION, for at least three weeks. If all is well at the end of that time try one of the onion family cooked and see if you get the same reaction. It is possible that because of cooking some foods are altered structurally and become acceptable.

Are there additives that appear to affect asthmatics more

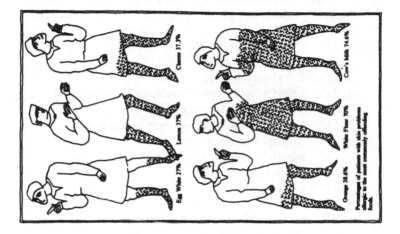

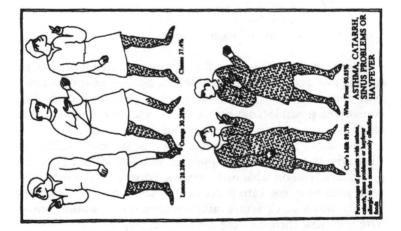

75

than others? I would say most certainly yes, but as there are over three thousand to choose from it is very difficult to be specific. Maurice Hanssen in his book *E for Additives* lists the following as possible triggers:-

E 212	Potassium benzoate
E 213	Calcium benzoate
E 214	Ethyl 4 hydroxybenzoate
E 215	Ethyl 4 hydroxybenzoate, sodium salt
E 216	Propyl 4 hydroxybenzoate
E 217	Propyl 4 hydroxybenzoate, sodium salt
E 218	Methyl 4 hydroxybenzoates
E 219	Methyl 4 hydroxybenzoate, sodium salt
E 310	Propyl gallate
E 311	Octyl gallate
E 312	Dodecyl gallate
621	Sodium hydrogen L-Glutamate
622	Potassium hydrogen L-Glutamate
623	Calcium dihydrogen di-Glutamate
627	Guanosine 5-(di sodium phosphate)
631	Inosine 5-(di sodium phosphate)
635	Sodium 5-Ribonucleotide

There are so many aspects of ingestants which it is necessary to take into account. It is possible that because of the benzoic acid contained naturally in banana and peas they could be considered possible 'triggers'. This is certainly not always the case and every person reacts differently to a stressor.

The safest and most sensible way is to find a Clinical Ecologist in your area and approach him for advice. He will give you advice on what to do, how to cope, and keep in touch with your progress. I stress yet again, there is no easy way out; if there was a quick acting tablet or potion that would eliminate the cause then the need for alternative procedures would be obsolete. There is no drug that completely eradicates the symptoms, the only way that can be achieved is by eliminating the cause.

CHAPTER 6

Depression; Pre-Menstrual Tension; and a note on Gut Conditions

DEPRESSION

Of all conditions, this is the most difficult: not for the practitioner but for the sufferer. It is human nature to feel sorry for someone who has a plaster on a limb or is paralysed, or has scarred features, but very few people have any patience with those who have a scarred mind. Unless someone has suffered the black despair on waking to another day, tummy rumbling and butterflies galore, legs shaking and so tearful, then it is not at all surprising that most sufferers are told to pull their socks up, pull themselves together or to grow up, whatever that is supposed to mean. I have had patients who have been afflicted from the age of three or four years of age. How do they grow up? What does it mean? Does it mean that they should not be so miserable and depressed, living in a black tunnel with no light at the end of it, that they should conform to what is considered the 'norm'? I have not met a depressive yet who would not rejoice at the thought of waking up to a day that held some excitement and normal emotions.

The awful truth is that many of you who do suffer from this condition need not necessarily do so. It is my experience that on numerous occasions it is the effect on the central and para-sympathetic nervous system created by a maladaption of the pancreas (allergy) that is often contributory to the condition.

It is a condition that has no specific 'triggers', but amongst the most implicated are: COFFEE, MILK, CHEESE, COLOURINGS and SUGAR.

I remember one man in particular who presented with a

manic depressive condition which had progressively worsened since he was in his teens. I shall call him John.

John was married to a German girl so there was certainly understanding that diet or extraneous factors could be contributory and that naturopathic or homoeopathic treatment could help. John had reached the point where he was afraid to go out and meet people. He had trained as a cabinet maker in this country and Germany. He was a clever man with his hands, but now these shaking hands let him down every time he picked up a piece of wood. He had been to his doctor and seen four specialists who diagnosed a depressive anxiety neurosis. He was told that therapy of various kinds might help but basically 'you must learn to live with it'.

As is often the case he came to see me as a last resort, saying 'I will try anything as long as I can start to live again'. I explained that all too often depressives could be affected by the foods they ingest; that the pancreas produces amino acids which are essential for correct mental function, and in his case this was not happening. These essential amino acids were not being produced in the right amounts and that by eliminating the cause his condition could improve. He became very interested and understanding the logic of the pancreatic reaction, excited at the prospect of leading a normal life. John was allergic to TEA, MILK, BUTTER, CHEESE, CHOCOLATE and WHITE FLOUR.

I explained that by eliminating he might well suffer considerable withdrawal symptoms and that for the first week he might well wish he had not embarked on the exclusion diet, but I was on the end of the telephone if he needed me, and to come back and see me in six weeks time. His next visit was unnecessary as his letter to me a few weeks later shows:

Dear Mr. Davies,

As you forecast to me when I visited you for the first time on Tuesday 19th April, I do not need the appointment booked for the 20th June.

A few weeks after dropping all Cows milk products, tea,

and white flour products from my diet, the chronic depression has gone!! As have also the pangs of anxiety and periods of feeling disturbed and troubled. A new feeling of confidence and contentment is being experienced daily. Also, physical improvements such as clearer skin, shinier hair and believe it or not, a clearer voice have been the result of your guide-lines. Only the stomach acidity is unfortunately still with me, but I expect that this will, too, in time disappear as did the other symptoms.

As useful 'side-improvements', I have also noticed that short-temperedness and irritability have all but vanished. It seems incredible that all these bad effects have been the result of wrong eating! But there you are – the proof is in the pudding!

If you are depressed take heart from this letter, realise that there is an alternative and consult a naturopath or homoeopath, preferably specialising in clinical ecology, and you may well be on the road to recovery.

PRE-MENSTRUAL SYNDROME

Menstruation is a natural event for women. Pre-Menstrual Tension is not. P.M.T. like all symptoms, are signals from the body that all is not right.

Typical Symptoms.

Mood fluctuation, depression, fatigue, headache, swelling and sensitivity of the breasts, oedema (water retention), backache, bloating, severe stomach pains.

How often, when couples come and see me together, has the husband said to me 'if you can stop the P.M.T. I shall be grateful, never mind the rest'. When P.M.T. rears its ugly head then a woman's job is a hundred times harder. How can a husband be expected to understand when his loving, cheerful, affectionate, calm and rational partner suddenly becomes a different woman?

It is an accepted medical fact that stress has an important part to play in P.M.T. Our bottom line defence against P.M.T. is providing ourselves with the sustenance we need to combat stress. Poor nutrition decreases our resistance to stress. Furthermore, poor nutrition or maladaption of controlling organs to digestion can even cause stress. What we eat can be either part of the solution, or part of the problem.

What are the logical steps to take?

PYRIDOXINE, vitamin B6 in the B vitamins is most associated with women's disorders. It has been used to treat P.M.T. since the early 1940s. B6 assists in the metabolism of oestrogen, restoring the oestrogen/progesterone balance. It is important for the normal functioning of the pituitary gland and for the metabolism of unsaturated fatty acids. Both of these activities affect the production of the sex hormones.

For many years I have used a naturopathic/homoeopathic preparation called AGNOLYT. It is the extracted juices of a native plant of the Mediterranean, vitex agnus castus. This also has the ability to balance the oestrogen/progesterone and consequently the majority of symptoms disappear within three months.

Evening primrose oil is also very beneficial in treating this complaint.

Those are the three major medicaments used to help with P.M.T. The other factor that seems to help enormously is to find the basic causatory triggers for the hormonal imbalance and eliminate these and a great majority of the symptoms disappear.

There are so many variables with this condition that I feel hard pressed to specify any one in particular. However it is amazing how often the 4C syndrome is contributory. Try eliminating COFFEE, CHEESE, CHOCOLATE, CITRUS and WHITE FLOUR and you may well find benefit.

In conclusion may I once again stress the importance of

consulting your doctor. Ask his advice: if he feels the condition is not one he can deal with, then consider the possibility of the available alternative.

GUT CONDITIONS
Diverticulitis – Crohns Disease –
Colitis – Spastic Colon

This is a distressing condition, which if not diagnosed and treated correctly can cause the sufferer's life to be dominated by one single thought: where is the nearest loo? Intermittent constipation and diarrhoea, stabbing pains in the gut, insatiable hunger that is never assuaged, complete revulsion to food or drink are a few of the classic symptoms; bloating after ingestion of food is another.

If you have seen your doctor and have had the necessary clinical investigation carried out with no success and the condition persists, then consider the possibility very seriously that it could be one of the foods or drinks that you ingest each day that may be causatory.

Sue had colitis, she was going to the loo as many as seventeen times a day, her weight had dropped from nine stone six pounds to seven stones three pounds. She had been through all the normal procedures and was still suffering every day. Sue was allergic to COFFEE, CHEESE, CITRUS, CHOCOLATE and WHITE FLOUR. 4C Syndrome? Migraine? Yes, I believe that Sue was suffering from a 'gut migraine': in many cases this does seem to be the case. However MILK is also a major contributory factor. By eliminating all of the above mentioned items you may well find that your condition improves.

At this point I would like to tell you of a 'phone call I had a fortnight ago. Mrs S.P. had come to see me eighteen months earlier with Crohns Disease. She was having as many as fourteen motions a day and her weight had dropped to 7 stone 3 lbs. After discovering her allergens the motions reduced to one or two a day and slowly but surely she recovered her normal weight, 9 stone 3 lbs. I had not heard from her for a long time until fourteen days ago and the conversation went something like this:

Mrs S.P.   Mr. Davies, I am sorry to trouble you but I had to call my G.P. last night as I was in such terrible pain and had diarrhoea and I don't know why.

G.H.D.   I am sorry to hear that, are you sure you did not ingest something?

Mrs S.P.   No, my diet has not altered for many months. I am too frightened to change things.

G.H.D.   Have you changed the brand of any of the products you use?

Mrs S.P.   Yes, I went to the health food shop last Friday afternoon and they had no Tomor margarine so I bought some Vitaquell, which you said was all right.

G.H.D.   My dear Mrs. P., that was a long time ago. In the last six months they have changed the contents of Vitaquell and added citric acid, and you are allergic to that.

Mrs S.P.   Gracious me, and I only had one slice at tea-time with it on.

G.H.D.   That is all you needed to create that reaction. Eliminate Vitaquell and let me know in a few days if things are no better.

I have not heard from Mrs S.P. for at least a fortnight. Be warned please! Check, check, and check again. Because a product is safe this week it does not mean it is safe forever. Your local health food shop is obviously a good place to shop but the staff do not have special training. Ask for advice by all means, but do not take all you hear as gospel. If you are in doubt, ask your practitioner.

Health food shops are often said to be expensive. I believe that in many instances they are; why on earth animal rennet-free cheese should be so expensive when the only difference is the rennet, I shall never understand; but many of the stores are now providing a good selection of wholefoods. In Great Britain many of the multiple retailers such as Boots, Sainsburys and Marks and Spencer now also have a good wholefood selection. Shop around, read labels and make sure you do not abuse your body by careless mistakes.

CHAPTER 7

Candida Albicans

CANDIDA ALBICANS – WHAT IS IT?

Candida Albicans is a yeast spore which lives in the mucous membrane of the gut in all of us from the age of approximately six months onwards. The gut flora should consist of 15% Candida Albicans approximately, the balance being made up by lacto bacillus acidophillus, lactobacillus foetidus and lactobacillus bifidus. Because it is present in all of us Candida Albicans tends to be overlooked totally by doctors seeking the cause of a certain condition. In some cases Candida proliferates to such an extent that notice does have to be paid to it, and instances of this kind have become more prevalent in recent years. Many explanations are offered for this proliferation; I believe that important contributory factors are the use of drugs (antibiotics, the pill, steroids) and the terrible over use of sugar in all our food. The over use of these has brought about a slow, insidious breakdown of the immune system and consequent proliferation of the yeast spores (Candida Albicans). When a healthy balance of foods is achieved, something which is not easy these days, a natural balance is maintained in the gut flora and the immune system has the ability to control and maintain homeostasis.

It is difficult when discussing a subject of this complexity not to become snowed under with technical terminology and lose the basic concept, in this case the destruction taking place within the body. I will endeavour not to do this and so couch these few paragraphs in terms that will mean something to anyone who has suffered the debilitating symptoms that can be experienced with Candida Albicans.

What are the symptoms?

Lethargy fatigue feeling under par
Vaginitis vaginal irritation and swelling
Throat soreness and irritation
Persistent irritating cough
Mouth infections of no specific origin
Skin conditions – acne and psoriasis
Depression
Anxiety states, tension and panic attacks
Menstrual and pre-menstrual problems
Prostatitis (inflammation of the prostate)
Loss of sexual libido
Constipation and diarrhoea

The immediate reaction to reading this list will be 'what is left?' These are conditions frequently experienced by most people and in minor cases clear up satisfactorily, only to appear in another form at a later date. You will also note, I am sure, that the symptoms I have mentioned are almost identical to those listed in previous chapters where 'allergy' is mentioned. What am I saying then, is that the symptomology of Candida Albicans is almost identical to that created by pancreatic malfunction. Yet again we are back to the instigatory organ of the endocrine and exocrine system. Only this time the simple expedient of eliminating the offending substances will not do. It is a matter of finding the correct supplementation of minerals and vitamins to help rebuild the immune system, resolve the balance in the gut flora, and ensure that the usual pitfalls of recovery are avoided: more on this later. You will also no doubt realise that the symptoms are indicative of a similar condition which has recently gained much publicity: M.E. (Myalgic Encephalomyelitis). I have treated this condition as Royal Free Disease for the last ten years with considerable success because I have treated it in the same way as Candida Albicans, and in every case I have treated there would appear to have been a pre-disposing Candidiasis.

If you have these symptoms and are concerned that it may be Candida, then the first and most obvious step to take is to consult your G.P. Not all G.P.'s are conversant with this problem, so do not be afraid to put forward the suggestion that it could be Candida Albicans. The next step from there should be tests to deduce whether this is the case or not. Do not feel disillusioned if the tests come back negative. This does often happen for a variety of reasons, the main one being that the condition is high in the transverse colon. If the symptoms persist then consult a Natural Health Practitioner of repute in your area. You should find that most are familiar with this problem and will be able to give you valuable advice. Should you still have problems after this step, then the only course you have is to consult a Clinical Ecologist who will deduce your allergens and in conjunction with correct diet and supplementation resolve the problem.

WHAT DIETARY MEASURES DO I TAKE?

The Candida Diet

Eat the Following Foods

Vegetables (I find parsnips can sometimes be a problem), Whole Grains (use only fresh supplies and organic where possible), Fish (I find bottom fish can sometimes cause reactions), Eggs, Meat, Poultry (if guaranteed antibiotic and hormone free), Cold pressed oils (especially olive oil for oleic acid content; not peanut or ground nut oil), Yoghurt (must be from antibiotic free source, plain only, goat or sheep milk), Fruit. Limit your intake of fruit, especially for the first few weeks. Fruit can carry mould and the natural sugar content can encourage Candida. Eat only fresh fruit, preferably picked and eaten on dry, low humidity days. Discover your tolerance for fruit by commencing with a peeled apple and then progress slowly once you are satisfied there is no reaction. In other words, keep the whole dietary regimen as simple and plain as possible for approximately three weeks. You should be seeing an improvement by then; if not you must consider the possibility that there may be a food sensitivity problem and the help of a Clinical Ecologist should be sought.

Do not take chances

It is a great temptation when on a rigid exclusion diet to have 'just a little'. You may be told by well meaning friends and relatives a little will not hurt. Please do not give in to the temptation or listen to the well meaning advice. If you were aware of the replication rate of Candida and how it can leave one debilitated for up to five days then you would know only too well that you cannot afford to take chances. No exclusion diet is cheap. You must be prepared for the extra expense, not only for the extra food that may be required but the supplementation that may also be necessary. Please note that I said supplementation and not drugs.

What should I avoid?

Yeast and all yeast products, marmite etc., mushrooms (fungii), fruit (in the initial stages), fruit juices, bread and all related products containing yeast, pizzas etc., margarines containing sugar or dextrose, alcohol (this includes cider), truffles, soya sauce, citric acid (nearly always a yeast derivative), citrus drinks – tinned or frozen, all malted products (cereals, sweets, or dairy products that are malted), all foods containing monosodium glutamate (often a yeast derivative), all vinegars, whether grape, malt or cider.

The following are either derived from yeast or contain elements that are:

Antibiotics, multi vitamin tablets (except when stated yeast free), B-complex vitamins (except when stated yeast free), selenium (as above), individual B-vitamins (as above).

Many alternative vitamin and mineral supplements are available which do not contain yeast, as most manufacturers are aware of the increasing problems associated with Candida Albicans. A lot of patients say they have difficulty in obtaining organic food products. Supplies should be getting easier all the time as supermarkets are providing at least some organic foods these days. If you are having difficulties then purchase the *Organic Food Guide* by Alan Gear, which is available from bookshops and health food shops.

Experience over the last two years has certainly proved to me conclusively that Candida Albicans can be corrected by the exclusion of yeast and sugar, the adoption of an allergy free diet and treatment with the various medicaments now available to health practitioners. It is worth mentioning in conclusion part of a treatise by a true and dedicated pioneer in this field, Doctor Renée Espy, called 'Candida Albicans – The Misdiagnosed Friend'. This is part of her treatise.

> At this time clinical research has shown that fungus is the body's S.O.S. Signal that it is immune deficient. After two and a half years of research fungus has proved to be a friend rather than something that needs to be destroyed. It has been found that the bacteria in the colon has been deficient and therefore unable to control fungal growth. Therefore it became necessary to find a way to stimulate bacterial growth without the side effects of a drug that would produce further side effects. This lead to the development of SPORE-X.
>
> I have used this product for the last six months and in nearly every case treated it has been effective. If any practitioner reads this and would like further information regarding this product then do not hesitate to contact me.

CHAPTER 8

M.E. (Myalgic Encephalomyelitis)

This has become a very 'popular' condition. Anyone with a penchant for feeling ill seems to climb onto the bandwagon, claiming a legitimate excuse for feeling ill, or wanting to feel ill. Hypochondriacs unite. A recent television programme on the subject was presented by an eminent and likeable woman doctor. In the past I have always had the greatest respect for this person. Her programmes were well researched and fairly presented. In this instance, sadly, this did not appear to be the case at all and she ridiculed the disease as psychosomatic. The programme was subsequently covered in the programme *Right to Reply* and Clare Francis and others replied in full.

I would like to ask what I think is an important question. Why create such publicity and devote millions of pounds of taxpayers' money to AIDS (Auto Immune Deficiency Syndrome) research and say so little about Myalgic Encephalomyelitis? The latter is recognised as being a Post Viral Fatigue Syndrome (PVFS), creating great physical and mental distress; is also recognised as being allergy related. When one comes down to basics, and after all that is the secret ingredient, we are talking about a BREAKDOWN IN THE IMMUNE SYSTEM.

Fabienne Smith in 'The Immune System: The Governing Factor in Health', Society for Environmental Therapy Newsletter, Vol 6, No 4, December 1986 states:

Non-Antibody Mediated Allergy:

It has been possible to show abnormal helper/suppressor cell ratios in people suffering from severe allergies. The same finding has also been established by various Clinical Ecologists in the U.S.A. It is also known that if the patient consumes foods or is exposed to chemicals to which he is allergic, the white blood cell population drops and remains lower than normal as long as the food continues to be eaten. Virus infections frequently seem to precipitate maladaptive allergic responses and inflammatory oedema during maladaptive food reactions causes local reduction in the oxygen supply in the tissues, leading to metabolic acidosis. Also hypoglycaemic episodes can be evoked in a person who has ingested any food, or come into contact with any chemical, to which he is allergic.

Whilst treating patients for Candida Albicans and Myalgic Encephalomyelitis (CA and ME), it has become increasingly evident that there is a great similarity between the two. It is amazing, when taking a case history, how the symptoms expressed by the patient can be related to either condition, and in many cases where Multiple Sclerosis is a factor, great similarities are noted. Needless to say no two patients have identical symptoms or allergies, due to lifestyle, eating habits or genetics. No two patients react in the same way to supplements and corrective remedies. No two patients have the same withdrawal symptoms. An MS sufferer reported to me that when he started Germanium his shaking (of the hands) stopped, his eyesight and his speech improved, but he was legless. A woman who started Germanium at exactly the same time reported no change in the condition at all, but she had started moving the big toe on her right foot for the first time in two years. Progress? Who can measure progress? I consistently stress to patients that only they can measure their success against what they were unable to do three, six or nine months ago.

M.E. (Myalgic Encephalomyelitis)

No one in his or her right mind would suggest that something so serious as a breakdown in the immune system can be overcome in a few weeks. That would be tantamount to a lie. It takes months and in some cases years for full recovery to take place.

WHAT ARE THE CAUSES?

Viral? Post Viral Fatigue Syndrome, Cytomegalovirus, Mononucleosis, Ebstein Barr Virus, Mixed Infection Syndrome, Defective Immunity Diseases. Wonderful labels, aren't they? But that is all they are you know – labels. Each one is a name attributed to a condition so that an immediate mental picture of the state a patient should be in attributable to that label can be formed. I must stress here again, as I will continue to do for the rest of my life, that you can hang labels on conditions until the proverbial cow comes home, but unless you find the causatory trigger, go back to basics, to pancreatic maladaption, you will never relieve the patient of those symptoms.

I intend to write in the near future another book which will deal in depth with Candida Albicans, Myalgic Encephalomyelitis and other labels that have been hung on people to pigeon hole them and in many cases give relief, because at least they have something that has a name, and no longer something that exists only in their minds. May God forgive any Doctor or Medical Practitioner who ever suggests that it is all in the mind as a possibility, without first establishing that every avenue has been explored.

You may well ask at this point why I am writing this section to *Overcoming Food Allergies* at all. The truth is of course that it is absolutely essential for you, the sufferer, to ascertain and endeavour to keep strictly to a cleansing diet, and to ensure that the supplementation taken is right for you as an individual. I so often hear Kyolic garlic mentioned as an aid to overcoming Candidiasis. I am sure that for those not allergic to milk this is so, but I have yet to find a patient suffering from Candidiasis or ME who can successfully tolerate milk in any shape or form. So, great care needs to be exercised. I would like to mention at this point something which is generally frowned upon by the G.P., and that is supplementation. Nutritional dietary advice is the primary objective and secondary to that is correct supplementation. No one who has an Immune Deficiency condition has got well without considerable supplementation. If the immune system is unable to support itself, then help must be given.

WHAT TYPE OF DIET?

The following suggestions should help to control the predisposing Candidiasis and strengthen the immune system.

Sunday
Breakfast – Home made muesli. Oats. Millet. Sunflower seeds. Pumpkin seeds. Flaked almonds. Mix thoroughly and use non sweetened soya milk.

Lunch – Omelette with onions, garlic and mixed salad. Use chinese leaves or organic lettuce. Peel cucumber. Scrape carrots. Use organic foods wherever possible.

Dinner – Roast lamb (cooked on a trivet) stuffed with garlic, greens, calibrese etc, carrots and roast potatoes. Use olive oil cold pressed for cooking. It is expensive but so is ill health. Do not use the meat juices for gravy. Use a home made vegetable stock. I have not found a suitable vegetable stock cube that meets all criteria.

M. E. (Myalgic Encephalomyelitis)

Monday

Breakfast – Scrambled eggs made with Tomor margarine. ORIGINAL Ryvita or high fibre rice cakes.

Lunch – Soup. Home made. Blanch celery, asparagus and onion family. Original Ryvita or rice crispbread.

Dinner – Left over cold lamb, potato, vegetables or salad.

Tuesday

Breakfast – Oatmeal porridge with bran (soya or oat) soya milk.

Lunch – Organic jacket potato with Tomor margarine and grated sheeps or goats cheese, do not heat or cook vegetarian cheese. Crushed garlic can be used.

Dinner – Brown rice or Basmati rice risotto with Tuna or salmon and mixed fresh vegetables.

Wednesday

Breakfast – Eggs (any way up). Ryvita or crispbread or oatcakes.

Lunch – Pilchards or mackerel in brine (no additives) and salad.

Dinner – Lambs liver (only use lamb) onions, garlic, brassicas, carrots and potatoes.

Thursday

Breakfast – Muesli and soya milk (as Monday)

Lunch – Vegetable or chicken soup (do not use the carcass) Ryvita or oatcake.

Dinner – Fried fish coated with egg and oatmeal. Use free flowing fish, not bottom fish at present. Chips and vegetables.

Friday

Breakfast	–	Porridge oats (see Tuesday)
Lunch	–	Cauliflower cheese (goat or sheep). Salad.
Dinner	–	Fishcakes. (Boiled cod, hake, halibut, haddock) mashed with egg to bind, herbs. Vegetables.

Saturday

Breakfast	–	Boiled egg. Ryvita or oatcake or rice cakes.
Lunch	–	Baked organic potato with salad.
Dinner	–	Stir fry basmati rice and diced vegetables topped with egg or fish of choice. Salad.

There will no doubt be raised eyebrows about the use of so many eggs, but when you are on a restricted diet, albeit temporarily, it is necessary to utilise the foods available and I have not had a patient come to any harm on this diet. It is not recommended for long terms and obviously there are some who will be allergic to some of the contents mentioned. The basic tenet is to use ORGANIC food whenever possible: free range eggs, free range chicken. You can always tell the difference between a commercial chicken and an organic chicken. The legs on a commercial chicken, when cooked, will fall off; the legs of the free range chicken will have to be pulled off! If you join the Soil Association (address at back of book) you can receive the Organic Growers and Suppliers guide, which is invaluable.

M. E. (Myalgic Encephalomyelitis)

WHAT SUPPLEMENTS DO I USE?

There are no definite rules to follow. Practitioners vary in their preference for a certain firm. Some have supplements made up to their own specifications and market them under their own labels. I will only say that you will need a good general vitamin/mineral supplement (yeast free) and after that it really is up to the practitioner to advise you on your additional requirements. You will certainly need something to balance up and replenish the gut flora. Spore-X, Pare-X, Uter-X, Lacto-Plus, C.L. Thymus, C.L. Liver etc. are all products from Nutri-West in the United States of America, available on prescription only. More generally available products could be obtained from Natures Best in the UK.

The Naturopath J. Hampton in his booklet 'Controlling Candida and ME with Earthdust' is a classic example of someone who has found what is best for him. He details in this booklet the procedures to follow and gives excellent advice to his patients.

LIVING WITH ALLERGIES

There will not be many people who read this book who, at some time or another, have not been told 'there is nothing more I can do, you will have to live with it'. YOU DO NOT HAVE TO LIVE WITH IT!!! The correlation between ME and CA is only the tip of the iceberg really. Most conditions bear some resemblance to these symptomatically, and it is certainly my experience, which is considerable, that providing you tackle the allergy problem in the correct way – cleansing the system from the inside with a correct detoxification programme – then good health will be a natural consequence. There will always be the basic causatory trigger, allergens, but once the immune system is repaired the peripheral allergens that have also shown up, and they can be many, will gradually resolve themselves and you will be left with only the basic allergens to cope with. The elimination of those is easy when the mind is clear and the body responding as it should. So take heart, it is not an insoluble problem, you are not on the scrap heap, help is available.

Remember what I said earlier. There is no better recommendation that by word of mouth. A patient who has been to a natural practitioner and has been treated successfully can make a recommendation which is truly worth having.

CHAPTER 9

Food Families

People who are allergic to a food often find that other foods in the same family affect them in the same way. Here is a fairly comprehensive list of food families for reference.

GRASS (Cereals)

1. Corn – cornstarch, cornflour, maize, maizemeal, corn oil, corn syrup, dextrose, glucose
2. Wheat – wheat flour, wholewheat and composite flours, gluten, wheat germ, cracked wheat, wheatstarch, bran
3. Barley – barley kernels, pearl barley, malt
4. Rye
5. Oats – porridge, oatmeals
6. Rice – ground rice, whole rice, brown rice, rice flour
7. Wild rice
8. Cane – sugar cane, molasses
9. Bamboo shoots
10. Millet – millet flour

SPURGE

1. Tapioca

MINT

1. Peppermint
2. Mint
3. Spearmint
4. Thyme
5. Marjoram
6. Savory
7. Basil and oregano
8. Sage

PINE

1. Juniper berries

CAROB

1. Carob bean
2. Carob powder

CHICORY

1. Chicory

PEPPER

1. Black pepper
2. White pepper

LAUREL

1. Avocado
2. Cinnamon
3. Bay leaves

MADDER

1. Coffee

POMEGRANATE

1. Pomegranate

GOURD (melon)

1. Pumpkin
2. Squash
3. Cucumber
4. Cantaloupe
5. Honeydew
6. Watermelon

MYRTLE

1. Allspice
2. Cloves
3. Guava

GRAPE

1. Grape
2. Raisin
3. Sultana
4. Cream of tartar

5. Vinegar

PINEAPPLE

1. Pineapple

BANANA

1. Banana

APPLE

1. Apple
2. Cider
3. Cider vinegar
4. Pectin (apple)
5. Pear
6. Quince

ROSE

1. Raspberry
2. Blackberry
3. Loganberry
4. Strawberry
5. Rose hip

GOOSEBERRY

1. Gooseberry
2. Blackcurrant
3. Redcurrant
4. Whitecurrant

BUCKWHEAT

1. Buckwheat
2. Rhubarb
3. Sorrell

CITRUS

1. Orange
2. Grapefruit
3. Lemon

4. Lime
5. Tangerine
6. Satsuma
7. Ugly fruit
8. **Angostura**

PLUM

1. Plum-prune
2. Cherry
3. Peach
4. Apricot
5. Nectarine, wild cherry & almond

GINGER

1. Arrowroot
2. Ginger
3. **Cardamum**

TEA

1. Tea

MAPLE

1. Maple syrup
2. Maple sugar

IRIS

1. Saffron

ORCHID

1. Vanilla

LILY

1. Asparagus
2. Onion
3. Leek
4. Garlic
5. Chives

GOOSEFOOT

1. Beet
2. Sugar beet
3. Chard
4. Spinach

LEGUMES

1. Navy beans
2. Lima beans
3. Kidney beans
4. String beans
5. Soya beans
6. Soya flour
7. Soya sauce
8. Soya lecithin
9. Lentils
10. Black-eyed pea
11. Peanut
12. Peanut oil
13. Peanut butter
14. Liquorice
15. Tragacanth
16. Gum acacia
17. Green pea
18. Field pea

MUSTARD

1. Mustard
2. Mustard greens
3. Cabbage
4. Cauliflower
5. Broccoli
6. Brussel sprouts
7. Rutabaga
8. Turnip
9. Kale
10. Radish
11. Watercress
12. Chinese cabbage
13. Horseradish

PARSLEY

1. Parsley
2. Parsnips
3. Carrots
4. Celery and celery seed
5. Celeriac
6. Caraway
7. Anise
8. Dill
9. Coriander
10. Fennel
11. Cumin
12. Angelica

ASTER

1. Lettuce
2. Endive
3. Artichoke
4. Dandelion
5. Salsify
6. Sunflower seed and oil
7. Sesame seed and oil

BIRD

1. Poultry – chicken, duck, turkey, goose
2. Game birds – pigeon, quail, woodcock, snipe, grouse and pheasant
3. Eggs

MELON

1. Melon
2. Courgettes
3. Marrow
4. Gherkin

PIG

1. Pork, bacon, pig products – ham, brawn, chitterlings, patés, sausages

MOLLUSCS

1. Snail
2. Squid
3. Mussel
4. Clam
5. Oyster
6. Scallop
7. Cockle

CRUSTACEANS

1. Prawns
2. Shrimp
3. Crayfish
4. Crab
5. Lobster
6. Scampi

SALT WATER FISH

Herring, sprat, anchovy, cod, sardine, bass, mackerel, sole, flounder, haddock, bream, coley, plaice, mullet etc.

FRESH WATER FISH

Perch, trout, salmon, pike, carp etc.

COW

1. Milk
2. Cheese
3. Yoghurt
4. Beef
5. Veal
6. Milk products

7. Butter

SHEEP

1. Lamb
2. Mutton

POTATO

1. Potato
2. Tomato
3. Egg plant
4. Red pepper–cayenne/ capsicum
5. Green pepper
6. Chilli
7. Belladonna
8. Tobacco

STERCULIA

1. Chocolate – Cocoa
2. Cola bean
3. Karaya gum

OLIVE

1. Olive (green)
2. Olive oil

BIRCH

1. Filbert nuts
2. Hazel nuts

FUNGUS

1. Mushroom

2. Antibiotics
3. Yeast

WALNUT

1. Black walnut
2. English walnut
3. Pecan

CASHEW

1. Cashew nut
2. Pistachio
3. Mango

PALM

1. Coconut
2. Date
3. Sago

BRAZIL NUT

1. Brazil nut

POPPY

1. Poppy seeds

NUTMEG

1. Nutmeg
2. Mace

MISCELLANEOUS

1. Honey

It is important to remember to rotate your foods each day if you are suspicious that a food allergen may be responsible for your condition. It does not always apply that because you are allergic to one item in a food family that you are necessarily allergic to them all. Either check them out yourself if you feel

...ᵤnt enough, or have them checked by your practitioner.

THE ROTATED DIET

A Rotated Diet is designed so that a food is eaten only every seventh day. This should enable you to pinpoint one group of .foods as being suspect for an allergic reaction. At a later stage you will be able to take the foods on separate days in a 'sliding diet', the individual food responsible should then be pinpointed.
This diet eliminates the most common allergens, cows milk, gluten containing grains, eggs, and stimulants such as coffee and tea.

If possible take all four foods at each meal, no drinks other than the juice of the day or water. All foods must be boiled in plain water, steamed, plain grilled, or cooked in the oven in a covered dish. No fats, gravies or oils are allowed. During the trial period it is essential that no other foods are ingested. Please remember that during the first week withdrawal symptoms may be felt, and at times they can be quite severe. In some cases it can be compared to a drug addict giving up the addicted drug, or an alcoholic giving up his booze.

Obviously a lot of imagination will be necessary to make the meals interesting but it can be done. Unfinished food from a particular day can be put in the freezer for the following week but please remember that frozen food is not as nutritious as fresh, and you should not rely on frozen food during the rotated diet or afterwards.

Once you have eliminated an offending food from your diet for six days, the reaction to the allergen on reintroduction may be fairly immediate and cause the return of one or more of your old symptoms, e.g. running or stuffed up nose, violent headache, a feeling of being bloated, extreme lethargy, bad temper, depression or extreme nervousness. The day that this reaction occurs mark it off on the diet sheet. In the third or fourth weeks, when it is certain which days these reactions occur, the change can then be made to the sliding diet so making it easy to identify the offending substance. If a mark has previously been made on a Tuesday and the Tuesday foods are underlined in red, when an adverse reaction occurs the 'red' food eaten on that day is the culprit. It is then possible to strike this food from the diet and substitute another for testing the following week.

Having worked out a basic diet of safe foods, it will then be possible to test the common allergens listed previously. At first it will be necessary to introduce only small amounts as the reaction may be quite severe. If the reaction is a bad one then take a teaspoon of bicarbonate of soda in warm water, this will help to alleviate the symptoms.

If you experience an adverse reaction then return to a safe diet for at least five days to allow the system to clear, then test for a suspect allergen again. After a few months it should be possible to identify all allergens in this way. Long and drawn out I am afraid, but the only safe way if you do not consult a practitioner. The rotated diet can be backed up by a supplementation of minerals and vitamins provided you are sure they are pure. Two companies that specialise in hypoallergenic preparations are Cantassium and Lamberts*.

EXAMPLE OF ROTATED DIET

MONDAY		TUESDAY		WEDNESDAY	
Turkey	1	Pork	2	Rabbit	3
Maize	1	Tapioca	2	Beans	3
Pear	1	Prunes	2	Grapefruit	3
Watercress	1	Cabbage	2	Green beans	3
Water		Prune Juice		Grapefruit juice	

THURSDAY		FRIDAY		SATURDAY	
Beef	4	Fish	5	Chicken	6
Potato	4	Banana	5	Buckwheat	6

Tomato	4	Pineapple	5	Apple	6
Lettuce	4	Spinach	6	Celery	6
Tomato juice		Pineapple juice		Apple juice	

SUNDAY
Lamb	7
Rice	7
Orange	7
Carrots	7
Orange juice	

FOLLOWED BY SLIDING DIET FOR THIRD WEEK

MONDAY		TUESDAY		WEDNESDAY	
Turkey	1	Pork	2	Rabbit	3
Rice	7	Maize	1	Tapioca	2
Apple	6	Orange	7	Pear	1
Spinach	5	Celery	6	Carrots	7
Apple juice		Orange juice		Water	

THURSDAY		FRIDAY		SATURDAY	
Beef	4	Fish	5	Chicken	6
Beans	3	Potato	4	Banana	5
Prunes	2	Grapefruit	3	Tomato	4
Watercress	1	Cabbage	2	Green beans	3
Prune juice		Grapefruit juice		Tomato juice	

SUNDAY
Lamb	7
Buckwheat	6
Pineapple	5
Lettuce	4
Pineapple juice	

BOOKS

Listed below are books you may find of great help if you have an allergy problem.

Allergies in Your Family: Doris J. Rapp M.D. Distributed in U.K. by Ward Lock Ltd, 116 Baker St. London W.1.

The Allergy Cookbook: Stephanie Lashford, Bath, Ashgrove, 1983

The Allergy Problem: Vicky Rippere, Wellingborough, Thorsons

Allergies – Your Hidden Enemy: Theron G. Randolph, Wellingborough, Thorsons. Probably the definitive work on allergies.

Brain Allergies – The Psychonutrient Connection: William H. Philpott M.D. and Dwight K. Kalita Ph.D. Available from Felmore Ltd. P.O. Box 1, Tunbridge Wells, TN1 1XQ £16.95

Chemical Victims: Dr. Richard Mackarness, London, Pan

Cooking for Your Hyperactive Child: June Roth. More than 200 artificial-additive-free recipes. Food sensitivity checklist with each recipe. Guide for identifying foods that contain 'hidden' allergens. Contact British Institute for Brain Injured Children, Knowle Hall, Bridgewater, Somerset.

E for Additives – The Complete E Number Guide: Maurice Hanssen, Wellingborough, Thorsons, 1984

How to control your Allergies: Robert Forman Ph.D., Larchmont

Medicines – A Guide for Everybody: Peter Parrish, Harmondsworth, Penguin

Not All in the Mind: Dr. Richard Mackarness, London, Pan

USEFUL ADDRESSES

UK

Action Against Allergy
43 The Downs
London S.W.20

British Migraine Association
Evergreen
Ottermead Lane
Ottershaw
Chertsey
Surrey

The Cantassium Company
Larkhall Laboratories
225 Putney Bridge Road
London SW15 2PY

Food Allergy Association
9 Mill Lane
Shoreham by Sea
West Sussex

Foodwatch
Butts Pond Industrial Estate
Sturminster Newton
Dorset DT10 1AZ

Foresight
The Old Vicarage
Witley
Godalming
Surrey GU8 5PN

Hyperactive Childrens Support
Group
59 Meadowside
Angmering
Sussex

National Society for Research
into Allergy
P.O. Box 45
Hinckley
Leicestershire
LE10 1JY

Sanity
77 Moss Lane
Pinner
Middlesex

Schizophrenia Association of
Great Britain
Tyr Twr
Llanfair Hall
Caernarvon
Gwynedd

Gwynne H. Davies, Clinical
Ecologist
Nirvana
Calway Rd.
Taunton TA1 3EQ
Tel (0823) 335610

USA

Allergy Foundation of Lancaster
County
Box 1424 Lancaster
Pennsylvania 17604

William J. Rea MD
8345 Wlnut Hill Lane
Suite 240
Dallas
Texas 75231

Ralph E. Smiley MD
8345 Walnut Hill Lane
Suite 240
Dallas
Texas 75231

Human Ecology Action League
 (HEAL)
505 North Lake Shore Drive
Suite 6506
Chicago
Illinois 60611

Alan Mandell Centre for Bio-
 Ecologic Diseases
3 Brush Street
Norwalk
Connecticut 06850

Society for Clinical Ecology
Del Stigler MD, Secretary
1750 Humboldt Street
Denver
Colorado 80218

Robert M. Stroud MD
8345 Walnut Hill Lane
Suite 240
Dallas
Texas 75231

Theron G. Randolph MD
505 North Lake Shore Drive
Chicago
Illinois 60611

Robert Cass, D.C.
Clinical Results
24000 Bessemer Street
Woodland Hills
California

APPENDIX

Percentages of patients with the condition noted who proved to be allergic to a number of commonly offending foods. The total number of patients (all conditions) included in the research was 2,728.

SKIN PROBLEMS
(Number included in Research 300)

Cow's Milk	74.60%
White Flour	70.00%
Orange	38.60%
Cheese	37.30%
Lemon	37.00%
Egg White	27.00%
Coffee	24.30%
Butter	23.30%
Egg Yolk	19.60%
Cocoa	14.60%
Food Colouring	13.30%
Tea	12.00%
Onion	10.60%
Goat's Milk	2.30%
Brown Flour	2.00%
Apple Skin	1.60%

ASTHMA, CATARRH, SINUS AND HAYFEVER
(Number included in Research 350)

White Flour	90.85%
Cow's Milk	89.70%
Cheese	37.40%
Orange	30.28%
Lemon	28.28%
Onion	26.28%
Butter	21.40%
Coffee	17.40%
Egg White	11.70%
Cocoa	10.57%
Tea	10.50%
Egg Yolk	10.00%
Food Colouring	8.57%
Brown Flour	3.70%
Apple Skin	2.85%
Goat's Milk	1.14%

ARTHRITIS
(Number included in Research 450)

White Flour	97.50%
Cheese	25.10%
Orange	22.40%
Cow's Milk	19.50%
Lemon	17.50%
Coffee	10.00%
Onion	9.70%
Butter	9.50%
Egg White	7.30%
Tea	5.50%
Cocoa	4.80%
Apple Skin	4.80%
Egg Yolk	4.60%
Food Colouring	1.50%
Goat's Milk	0.40%
Brown Flour	0.40%

MIGRAINE
(Number included in Research 228)

Cheese	84.60%
Coffee	77.60%
White Flour	67.10%
Cocoa	61.80%
Orange	60.00%
Lemon	59.20%
Cow's Milk	26.75%
Onion	25.00%
Tea	11.80%
Butter	9.60%
Egg White	8.77%
Egg Yolk	8.30%
Food Colouring	7.00%
Goat's Milk	2.60%
Apple Skin	2.19%
Brown Flour	0.87%

MULTI-FACTORIAL
(Number included in Research 1,400)

White Flour
Cheese
Cow's Milk
Coffee
Orange
Lemon
Cocoa
Onion
Butter
Egg White
Egg Yolk
Tea
Food Colouring
Apple Skin
Brown Flour
Goat's Milk